LIFE ON PURPOSE

LIFE ON PURPOSE

HOW LIVING FOR WHAT MATTERS MOST CHANGES EVERYTHING

VICTOR J. STRECHER

HarperOne
An Imprint of HarperCollinsPublishers

HarperOne

HarperCollins books may be purchased for educational, business, or sales promotional use. For information, please email the Special Markets Department at SPsales@harpercollins.com.

FIRST EDITION

Library of Congress Cataloging-in-Publication Data
Names: Strecher, Victor J., author.
Title: Life on purpose : how living for what matters most changes everything / Victor J. Strecher.
Description: First edition. | New York, NY : HarperOne, [2016]
Identifiers: LCCN 2015049467 (print) | LCCN 2016005572 (ebook) | ISBN 9780062409607 (hardback) | ISBN 9780062409676 (e-book)
Subjects: LCSH: Conduct of life. | Meaning (Philosophy) | Self-realization. | Life. | BISAC: SELF-HELP / Personal Growth / General. | HEALTH & FITNESS /
Healthy Living. | PSYCHOLOGY / Social Psychology.
Classification: LCC BJ1589 .S8737 2016 (print) | LCC BJ1589 (ebook) | DDC 158--dc23
LC record available at http://lccn.loc.gov/2015049467

16 17 18 19 20   RRD(H)   10 9 8 7 6 5 4 3 2 1

For Jeri

Contents

One

A HARBOR

1

CROSSROADS

I felt that what I was standing on had given way, that
I had no foundation to stand on, that that which I lived
by no longer existed, and that I had nothing to live by.

LEO TOLSTOY[1]

June 20, 2010, 5:15 a.m. In my kayak, a few miles from shore, paddling hard . . . Lake Michigan, smooth and ice-cold, my kayak cutting through a thick, silky curtain of water off the bow. Still in boxers and T-shirt, hadn't thought about dressing for the chilly morning air . . . wasn't really thinking.

I'd been woken by a dream, climbed out of bed, and a minute later pushed off into the lake. Not very smart—Lake Michigan owns hundreds of ships and certainly its share of puny kayaks . . . didn't really care.

Maybe I'll paddle to Wisconsin, I thought, but the sun stopped my paddling as it broke over the horizon. I turned toward the east and sat still . . . perfectly quiet.

Suddenly, a billion gold flecks of light surrounded me as the sun rose. In that moment, I felt the warmth and love of my daughter Julia.

Get over it, Dad, she was telling me. I almost tipped over. It was startling to hear her voice. She'd died just a few months before.

The crossroad of my life was right there—two miles off the shore of Lake Michigan. The signs were clear. One arrow said, "Change Everything." The other said, "Death." And Julia wasn't derisively telling me to "Get over it!" She was telling me that if I was to survive, I would need to *get over myself* and live for what matters most.

When I came back to shore, I realized it was Father's Day. This was her gift to me—the gift that would save my life.

Nineteen years earlier, Julia was born completely healthy. Then, when she was about six months old, she contracted the chicken pox virus. Rather than causing a few days of fever and rash, however, this virus attacked and destroyed her heart. No one knows why, but luckily, it happens to only a very small number of people. Unluckily, one of them was my daughter.

Her only hope, and it was a long shot, was a new heart; without it, she'd last only a few months. In 1990, very few children had received heart transplants, and there was almost no data on what would happen to them. Given this uncertainty, one of the biggest decisions we needed to make was whether to even put her on a transplant waiting list. The alternative was letting her die in peace.

As hard as it was even to think about this option, it was a very real consideration. We had no idea what would happen if she were to receive a new heart. No idea what the quality of her life would be. We were on the front edge of this wave of ice-cold water and would be for her entire life.

The discussions with family—my wife, Jeri, and older daughter, Rachael—were hardly idle dinner-table chatter. The topics were, "What is a good life?" and "What is a life worth living?" What if Julia died when she was three? How about nine? What about the quality of those years? Would we be happy with the decision we were making?

We decided to list her for a transplant. In part, frankly, we couldn't bear to let her die. But we were well aware that, if she did get a new heart, we'd need to work incredibly hard to keep her well—to give her a big life. We'd also need to approach life with her in a whole new way—in a way that assumed she might die at any moment.

When we talked about a "big life," we weren't referring to a "Make-A-Wish" life. Make-A-Wish is a nonprofit organization that provides extraordinary experiences for very sick and dying children. It's a wonderful group with a powerful mission—but we couldn't spend every day of Julia's life in Disney World. What we were determined to do was to provide her with a life of discovery, of meaningful relationships that extended beyond her family, and of love.

Julia received a new heart on Valentine's Day, 1992, and our lives were changed forever. She lived through many challenges and her life wasn't easy by any stretch, but it was a big life: friends, camp, softball, Girl Scouts, travel—experiences that many kids have but that Julia never took for granted.

This expression *took for granted* suggests that you're owed something, that you naturally deserve something. In this case, that life and its experiences should be *granted* to you. The unexpected thing that happened to the rest of our family is that we stopped taking our *own* lives for granted. We stopped expecting a certain life to happen to us and instead started creating our own lives. When this happened, our lives turned from black and white into Technicolor.

Personally, I started caring less about what people thought of me and more about what I thought of myself. As an assistant professor at a university, I started caring less about getting tenure and more about making a difference in the world. Most importantly, I stopped thinking that I'd live forever and started thinking that I'm on this earth for an extraordinarily brief period of time—so I should make the most of it.

Julia wanted to emulate the people who helped her so much through the years, so she enrolled as a student in the University of Michigan's School of Nursing. On spring break, 2010, we took our two daughters and their boyfriends to an island in the Caribbean. The third night of our stay, after having a dinner by the ocean, Julia turned to her boyfriend and said, "I'm so happy right now that I could die." And that night she did. She died, in her sleep, of a sudden heart attack.

The dreadful event that had been in the back of my mind for nineteen years had happened. Having considered this eventuality hundreds of times, I tried to gird myself. My goal would be to return to a normal, productive life. The question was just how long it would take: A week? A month? Six months?

A month later I was giving a talk to three hundred people on the topic of health and wellness—the subject of my profession. The audience knew nothing about my recent loss. The speaker before me was an occupational health physician who studied the impact of stressful events on workplace productivity. He said something like, "If you lose a parent, your productivity drops by an average of so-and-so percent, which returns in an average of such-and-such time. If you lose a spouse, your productivity drops by. . . ." Then he paused, took a breath, and said, "But if you lose a child, *your productivity never returns*."

He had no idea that I had just lost a child, but I still had a strong urge to tell him where he could shove his statistics. I didn't, but his words came back to me a few months later when I was sitting in my kayak, watching the sunrise. Would life ever be Technicolor again? Would I ever be productive again? Would I ever feel energetic again? Would I ever feel in control again? *Was there something I could do to get these things back?*

Those who lose their foundation to stand on often turn to Viktor Frankl, the Austrian psychiatrist. Frankl was one of the first—and certainly the foremost—to scientifically analyze the existential philosophy of purpose and meaning that can emerge from tragedy. In doing so, he created a new approach to psychotherapy.

Frankl observed through his personal experiences during three years as a prisoner in Nazi concentration camps that individuals who were able to maintain a purpose in their lives were more likely to survive: "Woe to him who saw no sense in his life, no aim, no purpose, and therefore, no point in carrying on. He was soon lost."[2]

The need to have a purpose in life is not only relevant to those who've suffered tragedy—it's relevant to everyone. And while Frankl's words have helped millions of people survive—and even grow from—the chaotic storms of life, many more millions have learned to simply live more purposeful lives. His famous work, *Man's Search for Meaning*, along with Julia's postmortem message to me on Lake Michigan became the clarion call to repurpose my life.

Viktor Frankl turned to philosophy for guidance as he developed his science of logotherapy ("meaning therapy"). As I began searching for a way to live after Julia's death, I also realized that the most helpful perspectives came from the world of philosophy.

Until that time, I'd been closed-minded to philosophy. It seemed irrelevant. The writings of Aristotle, Seneca, Kierkegaard and Nietzsche, Sartre and Camus, as far as I was concerned, were simply unreadable—period pieces with no relevance to my work or life. But after Julia died, their works seemed like letters written to me. They asked the big philosophical questions that concerned my daughter's life and my own: "What is a good life?" and "What is a life worth living?"

Beyond books, I started noticing people who seemed to have lives worth living. As a scientist in the field of public health, I have the privilege of working with many of these people. In 2003 an epidemic of the SARS virus started sweeping through major cities in China. Population sizes and densities in modern Chinese cities are immense compared with most other countries, and controlling the spread of this virus is extraordinarily difficult.

A few years ago I was visiting Tianjin's Centers for Disease Control and met with one of their senior public health professionals who worked in the city during the epidemic. China had instituted a complete quarantine of Tianjin. Only public health workers were allowed in—but not out. The death rate among these workers approached one in three. I asked him whether his family (who lived outside of the quarantine area) was concerned while he was in Tianjin. He smiled and said, "Of course!" What a stupid question. Did he fear for his own life? The smile dropped from his face, and looking me in the eye, he replied calmly, "This is what I do."

This was his purpose, what made his life worth living. The nineteenth-century philosopher Søren Kierkegaard wrote that "the thing is to find a truth which is true for me, to find the idea for which I can live and die."[3] This public health professional lived, and was willing to die for, his purpose. He saw many of his own colleagues die for their purpose. He ran into, not from, the threat.

I recently had lunch in Boston with another amazing person, Natalie Stavas, a pediatrician at Boston Children's Hospital. Natalie's life changed when, within eight hundred yards of finishing the 2013 Boston Marathon, she heard a second loud explosion near the finish line. She'd heard the first blast and mistook it for celebratory fireworks. The sounds of the second blast and the screams changed her mind. Spurred by shouts of "Sniper!" and "Terrorists!" and "Bombs!" most people were running away from the blast area. Natalie ran (remember, she'd just run twenty-six miles!) *toward* it.

Despite direct orders from a policeman not to cross the race barriers, Natalie jumped them to reach and treat four victims. One died; the other three survived. She still tears up as she remembers the one she couldn't save. Hailed as a hero by the president of the United States among many others, she still feels that her actions were nothing particularly special—they were simply a reflection of who she is.

Seated in the back of a plane recently, Natalie became aware that a man in first class was choking and couldn't breathe. She shot out of her seat and ran to the front of the plane, popped the food from his throat, and got thrown up on. After Natalie returned soggily to her seat in coach, the passenger next to her seemed shocked that she'd so readily launch herself into action. It's just *who she is*, she thought.

As we'll see in what follows, if Natalie doesn't get blown up or puked on too much, she'll likely live longer than she would if she *didn't* run toward scary things. More importantly, she will live *better*. Mark Twain once said that a "man who lives fully is prepared to die at any time." The Tianjin public health worker and Natalie Stavas seem prepared to die at any time. No doubt they're also more fun to hang out with at parties.

THE RESEARCH

In research studies, purpose in life is usually measured with statements such as, "I have a sense of direction and purpose in life," and "Some people wander aimlessly through life, but I am not one of them." Respondents then typically assess the statements using scales that range from one to seven, and the responses to each statement are combined to form an overall index of purpose.

Studies using these measures demonstrate that people reporting a strong purpose in life, on average, live longer lives than those with a weak purpose. A recent study[4] following over seven thousand middle-aged American adults for fourteen years found that even a one-point increase on a seven-point scale of purpose resulted in an over 12 percent reduced risk of dying. This result wasn't conditional on the person's age or whether they'd retired. Importantly, general measures of happiness or sadness did not influence risk of death, nor did they affect the impact of purpose in life.

I spend my days at work studying factors that make us healthy or unhealthy. Together, tobacco use, a poor diet, inactivity, stress, and other lifestyle factors contribute to roughly half of disease and early death.[5] The media is filled with messages about these issues, but far less is written about lack of purpose in life; yet, based on current evidence, it contributes at least as much to disease and death as do these other factors.

So let's look at other evidence testing the benefits of having a strong purpose in life. In a study[6] of over 1,500 adults with heart disease followed for two years, every one-point increase on a six-point purpose-in-life scale resulted in a 27 percent lower risk of suffering a heart attack. In a study[7] of over 6,000 adults followed for four years, every one-point increase on a six-point purpose scale resulted in a 22 percent reduced risk of a stroke.

These aforementioned studies began with large cohorts (groups) of people. Researchers measured lots of things about these people, such as their age, gender, diet, physical activity, weight, smoking behavior, existing medical conditions and disease, and many other factors. They then followed the cohorts, measuring outcomes of interest years later. Who lived and who died? Who got sick? How many health-care services did they use? Were the measures initially collected associated with these outcomes?

In public health, as in other sciences, great pains are taken to avoid mistaking correlation for causation. That means that when studying potential risk factors, it's essential to statistically control for other factors that might actually be causing changes in the outcomes of interest. For example, if researchers are looking at the effects of cigarette smoking, it might be that people with lower education, lower income, or poor health practices are also more likely to smoke and that it's those factors that cause the health trouble. Controlling for these factors gives us more confidence that the risk factor we're studying is the one responsible.

The same principle holds true when studying the link between purpose in life and mortality, heart attack, or stroke. In each of those studies, the researchers controlled for a broad spectrum of other factors that might have been responsible for the associations.

Let's look at another outcome many people are terrified of: Alzheimer's disease. At the Rush Alzheimer's Disease Center, Patricia Boyle and her colleagues[8] followed over nine hundred seniors for seven years, looking for the incidence of Alzheimer's. The results were startling. Over that period, seniors with a low purpose in life were 2.4 times more likely to develop Alzheimer's disease than those with a high purpose in life. In a separate study,[9] the same research team found a slower progression of the disease among those who developed Alzheimer's and had a high purpose in life.

People with a strong purpose in life also, on average, do better psychologically and socially than those without. They have better sex,[10] sleep better,[11] are less likely to become depressed,[12] and are more relaxed.[13] Diabetics with a strong purpose are more likely to have their blood glucose under control.[14] People who have received drug and alcohol rehab are half as likely to relapse six months later if they started treatment with a strong purpose.[15]

Physiologically, purpose in life is associated with an increase in natural killer cells that attack viruses and cancerous cells.[16] Purpose is also associated with a reduction in inflammatory cell production (which we'll discuss in the next chapter)[17] and an increase in HDL ("good") cholesterol.[18]

Do these outcomes translate into reductions in health-care costs? My colleagues Eric Kim, now at Harvard University, and Carol Ryff from the University of Wisconsin and I studied the impact of purpose in life on health-care utilization among over seven thousand adults followed for six years.[19] We found that, after statistically controlling for initial demographics, health behaviors, and health status, every point improved on a six-point purpose-in-life scale resulted in a 17 percent reduction in nights spent in the hospital. If you had a purpose of five on a six-point scale, you'd have an average of 36 percent fewer hospital nights per year than a person who had a purpose of two. I know of no other lifestyle behavior that produces this effect on health-care use.

Lately, one of the most famous researchers in the world has studied the impact of life purpose. Elizabeth Blackburn, the 2009 Nobel Prize winner in medicine, discovered the role of telomeres, which are located at the end of our chromosomes and act a bit like the aglets (plastic caps) that keep shoelaces from fraying. When our telomeres shorten, our chromosomes are more susceptible to damage, and we're more likely to get sick.

Over a decade ago in her research with Elissa Epel and other colleagues,[20] Blackburn studied mothers with chronically ill children and found that the mothers' telomeres were shorter by at least one decade of life than mothers without sick children. She and her colleagues suspected that this telomere shortening was due to the stresses of caring for a sick child.

Meditation has been shown to reduce stress, so Blackburn and her colleagues[21] created an experiment that randomly enrolled some subjects in a three-month meditation program, and others to a waiting list for the program. The study sought to determine whether meditation would reduce stress, which might, in turn, increase an enzyme called telomerase that fuels telomeres.

They found that the meditators, when compared with the control group, did indeed have more telomerase. What they also found, however, was that the meditators were developing a stronger purpose in their lives, and *it was the purpose in life, not the meditation,* that was associated with higher levels of telomerase.

IF PURPOSE WERE A DRUG

So let's imagine a drug that was shown to add years to your life; reduce the risk of heart attack and stroke; cut your risk of Alzheimer's disease by more than half; help you relax during the day and sleep better at night; double your chances of staying drug- and alcohol-free after treatment; activate your natural killer cells; diminish your inflammatory cells; increase your good cholesterol; and repair your DNA. What if this imaginary drug reduced hospital stays so much that it put a dent in the national health-care crisis? Oh, and as a bonus, gave you better sex?

The pharmaceutical company who made the drug would be worth billions. The inventors of the drug would receive Nobel Prizes and have institutes named for them!

But it's not a drug. It's purpose. And it's free.

Oh, and the side effects? More friends. More happiness. Deeper engagement in life. And did I mention better sex?

My initial interest in research studying purpose in life was triggered by a personal experience—the loss of my daughter Julia. I found a clue on Lake Michigan in my kayak when I felt her telling me that I needed to get over myself, my "ego." Then I found comfort in knowing that I wasn't alone, that in fact philosophers had been examining questions of life purpose for thousands of years and that these big questions are now, for the first time in history, being studied using the methods of science.

So far so good. But we're only at the first step in our understanding. As we walk down this path, we'll find many important questions to explore: Why does having a strong purpose in life protect us from illness? How do we find our purpose in life? Does it matter what the purpose is? How do we align our lives with this purpose? Come to think of it, what do we even mean by "purpose in life"?

So as Julie Andrews sang, let's "start at the very beginning" . . . with philosophy.

2

ORIGINS OF PURPOSE

Begin discussion—by saying what is happiness.

CHARLES DARWIN[1]

OCTOBER 20, 2014, 10:15 A.M. BOARDING THE PLANE IN FRANKFURT, Germany, I was thinking about an upcoming Purpose in Life presentation I was giving that afternoon in London. The slides weren't quite finished, as I was struggling with one particular section, which I called the "science of philosophy."

I'd recently read Stephen Hawking's book *The Grand Design*[2] and was stopped cold by something he wrote in the very first paragraph: *"Philosophy is dead."* He was pointing out that philosophers and religious leaders have misled human beings for thousands of years. When it came to our physical laws, the ancient philosophers, like Socrates and Aristotle,[3] seemed to just make stuff up. Hawking points out that even basic methods of *testing* their assertions seem to have eluded them.

The ancient world's belief in whatever really smart old men with beards had to say because, well, they were really smart old men with beards got us into a lot of trouble. Just ask Galileo, who, while also being a really smart old man with a beard, took the trouble to put his assertions to the test. He was rewarded by being put on trial by the Church's Inquisition. Hawking was saying that nonscientific methods perpetuated ignorance and needless misery through the centuries and that their day was mercifully over.

A like-minded scientist, Lawrence Krauss, is an astrophysicist known for his work on the origins of the universe. He also doesn't seem to mind, well . . . *stirring the pot*. I have an amateur interest in astrophysics and in Krauss's work and was reading a statement he made in a public debate with a philosopher:

"The chief philosophical questions that do grow up are those that leave home."

What does this statement mean? Lawrence Krauss was saying that the big questions can't really be answered by philosophers—they can only be asked. It takes the methods of science to answer them. So Krauss was telling philosophers to create their big questions, nurture them, raise them to maturity, then let them find their way in the real world. The world of science.

The day before my flight I'd created a slide featuring a picture of Lawrence Krauss along with his quote and was trying to work it into my London presentation. I generally agreed with Krauss and Hawking that scientific method was necessary to test big questions. The problem I saw in the hectoring from both of them was that the "hard sciences" seem to take a pass on many of our biggest questions. The function of your left-handed amino acids? Fascinating! The function of your leftover years after retirement? Yawn.

With the roughly three trillion miles I fly each year, I was able to turn left as I entered the jumbo airplane, into a huge, nearly empty first-class section. *Ah,* I thought. *The whole plane to myself! I'll have hours of uninterrupted time to work Krauss's antagonistic statement into my talk.*

I then realized that my assigned seat was next to the *only* other person in the entire cabin. A bit miffed, I thought as I was sitting down that I'd move to another seat after the flight took off. Leaning over to shove my briefcase under the seat, I noticed in the open case next to mine a book about the universe: it was by Lawrence Krauss. *Wow,* I thought. *That's an amazing coincidence! Maybe I'll stay in this seat and see what this guy thinks of Lawrence Krauss.* I turned and looked up at the briefcase's owner. It was Lawrence Krauss.

Over 2,300 years ago, Aristotle posed one of *the* big philosophical questions: *What is the ultimate purpose of human activity?*

Aristotle concluded that the ultimate purpose of human activity is *happiness*. Did he scientifically test this assertion? Not that we know of, though in fairness, they didn't have large epidemiological cohorts, randomized trials, complex statistical forecasts, functional magnetic resonance imaging, or genomic and epigenetic assays in 300 B.C.

Yogi Berra once said that "you can observe a lot by just watching." And Aristotle watched more than his share. He was a student of Plato and a teacher of Alexander the Great.

Let's stop here just for a second.

Aristotle taught Alexander the Great. Picture yourself with Alexander as he's wondering whether to invade, oh . . . let's say India.

Aristotle observed virtues and vices that we couldn't imagine in our modern era and maintained that, unless we were a slave, we choose for ourselves the kind of life we live. In psychology, the capacity for human beings to make these kinds of choices and to impose those choices on the world is called "agency." Though this seems obvious to most people today—that individuals have at least some agency—it was quite different in Aristotle's time, when it was the norm to make sacrifices to the gods to influence one's fate.

In the *Iliad*, Homer's ancient epic poem, an archer loses a shooting competition not because of his own performance but because he failed to sacrifice one hundred lambs to the god Apollo, who apparently holds grudges. Another archer does make a sacrifice of one hundred lambs to Apollo and wins the contest. (Thousands of years later, this tactic would come to be known as "working the refs.")

Consider for a moment how this mind-set might influence your behavior in the modern era. Before you drive to work, you might toss into your Costco sacrificial fire pit a package of frozen chicken breasts to assure a safe commute. If your fate was determined by the gods, you might not care that much about *actually driving safely*—a point made vividly clear when I was a child in Sunday school and our minister would drive us in his car at over ninety miles per hour. "If God wants us to die, we'll die. If he wants us to live, it doesn't matter how I drive!" We in the backseat, of course, loved our minister's approach to life and to driving. Our parents, oddly, did not. He didn't stay around long.

Without a sense of personal agency, people throughout history would sacrifice anything they could round up—including, at times, their own children. If you live in a chaotic environment, you still try to maintain control—even if it's not by your personal agency. Aristotle's approach to living changed the way people thought about cause and effect, heralding in Western civilization.[4] The beginning of human agency.

If we do have agency, Aristotle considered, we should be thoughtful, using the gift of reason, in choosing what to be in our lives. One of the most delightfully dark statements of our own agency is from the writer Kurt Vonnegut, who said that "we are what we pretend to be, so we must be careful about what we pretend to be."[5] Aristotle thought that, with a few exceptions, we decide what we become.

Back on the plane, I exclaimed, "You're Lawrence Krauss!" Since Lawrence Krauss already knew that he was Lawrence Krauss, he seemed unsurprised by this statement. He did, however, seem somewhat concerned that the last person in the world he'd want to have sitting next to him had just sat down next to him. He acknowledged that he was indeed Lawrence Krauss. I opened my computer, clicked to my slide of him, and said, "I'm afraid I have a bone to pick with you, Lawrence Krauss. You may want to take another seat before we take off."

TWO KINDS OF HAPPINESS

So if the gods, fate, luck, or chance aren't solely responsible for our outcomes—if we indeed have human agency—where do we turn to make the right decisions? Socrates, the Athenian street philosopher, famously said that "the unexamined life is not worth living." As he was teaching others to examine their lives, Socrates would often stop in the middle of a conversation, leaving briefly to consult his inner self. When he returned, he would speak with the confidence that he was conveying truth.

Sculptors of his era would occasionally hide a golden figurine inside terra-cotta busts they made of the Greek gods. One of Socrates's students likened him to one of these statues. On the outside he was a bald, potbellied man. His inner self, however, was godlike, and Socrates was considered by his students (including Plato) to be in touch with his true self.[6]

Aristotle used an odd word to describe the connection with the true self: *eudaimonia.* In this word is the term *daimon,* which means the "true" and "most divine."[7] The Greeks thought that every person had an inner daimon and that we should find and live in harmony with it. The concept of a true self that transcends one's ego-focused desires is found in many Western and Eastern religions as well as in more modern psychological approaches.

The happiness attained by the *self-transcending* state of eudaimonia, Aristotle asserted, may be contrasted with *self-enhancing* "hedonia," which as you might expect, concerns hedonism, the pursuit of pleasure derived from gratifying short-term desires. He understood that we all seek hedonic pleasure, but unlike many of his fellow philosophers (such as Epicurus), he warned against the excess of it, stating, "The many, the most vulgar, would seem to conceive the good and happiness as pleasure. . . . Here they appear completely slavish, since the life they decide on is a life for grazing animals."[8]

We don't consider ourselves grazing animals, but most of us do like to graze: on good food, drink, sex, beauty, and other things that give us pleasure. And yet most of us still understand that there's more to life than just pleasure. If Aristotle were alive today, he might counsel, "Listen to your heart and don't act like Charlie Sheen." We might agree, but when we use the term *happiness*, we don't typically think about happiness derived from eudaimonia.

We've reduced our definition of happiness to the dopamine-driven experiences of pleasure. Eudaimonia sounds like a bit more work. And do we really have time to consult our "inner daimon"—to explore the direction we're taking in our lives? The philosopher David Norton asserts that "most of us today have no sense of an oracle within. . . . Turning our backs to the void, we become infinitely distractible by outward things, prizing those that 'demand' our attention. We secretly treasure the atmosphere of world crises, for the mental ambulance-chasing it affords. Meanwhile we armor ourselves with mirrors to deflect the inquiring eyes of others."[9]

Consider this in your own life: Are you "distractible by outward things"? Most of us understand this in reference to material objects, but I find it interesting that Norton also refers to the crisis of the week. How many conversations have you had that turn into little more than a parroting of the calamities described on National Public Radio or (with more conservative friends) Fox News? Chilean coal miners? An avalanche? Hurricane? Beheading? It's not that these events are unimportant, but as Norton points out, this "mental ambulance-chasing" distracts us from a careful examination of ourselves—our inner daimon makes us uncomfortable because we're terrified that it will tell us that we're heading in the wrong direction.

On the plane, Lawrence Krauss unconvincingly told me he'd be happy to stay in his seat next to me and discuss the bone I had to pick with him regarding his claim that the big questions had to leave their philosophical homes for the world of science.

"I agree," I said. "The big philosophical questions must leave home but then receive proper attention from science. They need to find a job so they don't have to move back with their parents!"

Science needs to study these big questions so they don't linger for centuries in philosophical limbo. Krauss seemed to enjoy the forced meeting and was open to my point.

One could argue, as Krauss does, that philosophy lets us down by not sufficiently answering its own questions. But science also lets us down by not addressing the big questions or helping people apply the answers in their daily lives. Until recently. Over the past decade, scientists have begun studying the impact of hedonia and eudaimonia on our health and well-being.

That's right—scientists are now exploring one of the biggest philosophical questions in history. Here are three such explorations:

In 2013, psychologist Barbara Fredrickson led a team of researchers "to map the potentially distinct biological effects of hedonic and eudaimonic well-being." The "biological effects" they were looking at were the expression of genes that were either good or bad for us.

We can respond to stressful conditions with more antiviral agents and antibodies (good for us) or with inflammation (bad for us). The type of response, however, varies between individuals. So what is it about individuals that causes this response to vary? Fredrickson thought it might have something to do with Aristotle.

In her study, healthy adults first completed a questionnaire measuring levels of hedonic and eudaimonic well-being. Hedonic questions assessed desire-driven happiness, whereas eudaimonic questions assessed purpose and meaning, growth-related challenges, and contribution to society.[10] They then filled out a questionnaire measuring depressive symptoms and provided blood samples to assess gene expression.

Here's what Fredrickson's team found. First, hedonia and eudaimonia were connected; if you were hedonically well, you were more likely to also be eudaimonically well, and vice versa. Both modes of happiness were also associated with lower levels of depression. So far, this suggests that there either is no difference between hedonia and eudaimonia or that their effects are similar.

What turned heads was the finding from the blood samples. Participants scoring high on the *hedonic* scale were far more likely to have inflammatory gene expression and decreased expression of genes involved in antibody and antiviral response, whereas participants scoring high on the *eudaimonic* scale had the *opposite* pattern of expression. In other words, participants with greater eudaimonia were physiologically healthier.

As the researchers state, "Hedonic and eudaimonic well-being were originally distinguished to resolve basic and ancient philosophical questions regarding the best way for humans to live. The present data offer little grounds to prefer one mode of happiness over the other based on affective experience, but they identify a stark contrast at the level of molecular physiology."

But before we assume that Angelina Jolie will live to be 140 and Paris Hilton will explode in a giant ball of pus, we should do what scientists like to do when something as radical as this is found: more research.

Aristotle stated that eudaimonia is found more among those who have "kept acquisition of external goods within moderate limits" and that "any excessive amount of such things must either cause its possessor some injury, or, at any rate, bring him no benefit."[11] Christopher Niemiec and his colleagues[12] were interested in whether eudaimonic versus hedonic aspirations of individuals just beginning their careers had an influence on well-being. In a study of graduating college students, the researchers found first—perhaps unsurprisingly—that they were more likely to attain what they aspired to. Those placing importance on money, fame, and image (hedonic) were more likely to attain them, while those who aspired to greater personal growth, relationships, and community (eudaimonic) were more likely to attain these outcomes.

Those who attained hedonic aspirations, however, reported greater anxiety and physical symptoms of poor health, whereas those attaining eudaimonic aspirations reported greater life satisfaction, self-esteem, and positive feelings.

In my own thirty years of teaching, I've noticed a similar pattern: students with eudaimonic aspirations are generally happier in the long run, even in terms of career success. In the short run, they tend to be better students, being more engaged in the substance of their classes as opposed to simply working for a grade. They're interested in mastering the course material, and this often translates into a successful and meaningful career.

That said, one might wonder whether students who endorsed eudaimonic aspirations weren't simply better at answering questions in a way they thought would please the researchers. Could these students have greater well-being because their brains are better at telling people what they want to hear?

Studying people's brains more directly can give us insights that questionnaires and self-reports sometimes miss. We send oxygen to the sections of our brains that are being used the most. Encounter a rattle-snake while hiking, for example, and more oxygenated blood immediately flows to a part of the brain that generates a fear response. Before you know it—literally—you jump back.

Hear the sound of an ice cream truck and more oxygenated blood is likely to immediately flow to your ventral striatum, a part deep in the brain that's associated with rewards. But individuals *vary* in their brain's response to different possible rewards, which can be measured by the amount of oxygenated blood flowing to the ventral striatum. Using this strategy, scientists can determine whether the sound of an ice cream truck is more rewarding to you or to me.

So do we vary in our neural responses to eudaimonic versus hedonic rewards, and if so, what difference does it make?

In a recent study,[13] researchers examined activation in the ventral striatum of adolescents when engaged in eudaimonic versus hedonic decision making. The adolescents' brains were scanned using functional magnetic resonance imaging (fMRI) while making eudaimonic decisions to *donate* money to others or hedonic decisions to *keep* the money. Adolescents who had more blood flow to the ventral striatum during eudaimonic versus hedonic choices could then be identified. In addition, the researchers measured symptoms of depression in the beginning of the study and one year later.

Sure enough, some adolescents' reward systems responded to the eudaimonic choices, whereas others' responded to hedonic choices. The bigger question was whether this difference in reward response had an influence on depressive symptoms. The results were clear. After a year, adolescents with greater activation of their brain's reward system while giving money had, on average, a *decline* in depressive symptoms, whereas those with greater activation in this system when keeping the money had an *increase* in depressive symptoms.

In fMRI, under the controlled situation created by the researchers, the adolescents didn't have control over the activation of different parts of their brains—that is, the adolescents couldn't manipulate their results to please the researchers. This further confirms that eudaimonic and hedonic forms of happiness are indeed different and that they produce very different effects.

PURPOSE IN LIFE

So what is the ultimate purpose of human activity? Is it just being nice? No. Eudaimonia requires self-discovery: Of the things you care most deeply about and that transcend your immediate desires. Of the people you most want to emulate. Of the legacy you want to leave. Of your purpose in life. Of the habitual actions leading to the fulfillment of this purpose. This process may be likened to leaving your old town and embarking on a journey. You jump into your boat and sail into a new, uncharted sea, toward a better harbor.

As Lawrence Krauss and I were getting off the plane in London, I asked him what he was working on. He replied that he was studying how the universe emerged from nothing. Oh. Lawrence Krauss is, indeed, taking a big philosophical question and giving it a job—in the realm of science. I had no further bone to pick with him. Going through customs he offered me a ticket to the London premier of *The Unbelievers*, the movie in which he costars with prominent atheist Richard Dawkins.

When the John Templeton Foundation[14] (whose motto is "Investing in the Big Questions") asked Krauss, "Does the universe have a purpose?" he replied, "Unlikely." He then went on: "A universe without purpose should neither depress us nor suggest that our lives are purposeless. Through an awe-inspiring cosmic history we find ourselves on this remote planet in a remote corner of the universe, endowed with intelligence and self-awareness. We should not despair, but should humbly rejoice in making the most of these gifts, and celebrate our brief moment in the sun."

Interestingly, Aristotle's name means "best purpose." So what do you say we jump in our boats, make the most of our gifts, find the best purpose we can, and, in the words of my accidental seatmate, celebrate our brief moment in the sun?

3

OUR BEST PURPOSE

My purpose is to help others create a purpose in their lives, to teach every student as if they were my own daughter, to be an engaged husband and father, and to enjoy love and beauty.

VICTOR J. STRECHER

When he was nine years old, the future composer Samuel Barber wrote a letter to his mother declaring his purpose in life: "to be a composer, and will be I'm sure." To this he added, "Don't ask me to try to forget this unpleasant thing and go play football. Please."[1] Obviously, some know early in life what they're born to do; others spend their entire lives without a purpose. Some may have one but be unable to articulate it.

Here are some purposes of well-known and not-so-well-known individuals:[2]

"To be *The* Tenor Saxophonist"—Dexter Gordon (jazz saxophonist).

"To contribute something meaningful back to the whole of society, to alleviate world hunger, to make the world a better place for those yet unborn, to build an everlasting peace throughout the world"—Gary Lamb (farmer).

"To keep trying to understand a little more deeply the universe we are all in, to try to take one more step on this unending quest. And to have fun along the way"—Ronald Graham (theoretical mathematician).

"To relieve suffering and to exercise compassion. We are all in this together, for life is a common, not an individual, endeavor"—Harry Blackmun (U.S. Supreme Court justice).

"To make a dent"—Studs Terkel (author, *Hard Times*).

"To put a ding in the universe"—Steve Jobs (cofounder, Apple).

"To live fully, experiencing each moment, aware, alert and attentive. We are here, each one of us, to write our own story—and what fascinating stories we make!"—Madeleine L'Engle (author, *A Wrinkle in Time*).

"To express solidarity with the poor and try to change their situation"—Gustavo Gutierrez (Peruvian Catholic priest).

Not all purposes are so lofty and motivating; some have a certain funky charm of their own. Jose Martinez, a taxi driver, responded to the question with, "To die, just live and die. I live driving a cab. I do some fishing, take my girl out, pay taxes, do a little reading, then get ready to drop dead . . . Life is nothing."

I take a lot of cabs, and often strike up conversations with the drivers. I occasionally ask them whether they have a purpose in life. Their surprising, often moving answers blow me away again and again: "I'm here in this country, working twelve-hour days, to provide a future for my children. They'll be the first ones in our family to ever go to college." I relate these stories on the first day of class each winter semester at the University of Michigan, and invariably some of my first-generation college students come up to me afterward, telling me about their parents who worked like this to get them into college.

Children who have gone through difficult situations, from being very sick to being bullied or abused, often enter college with a strong purpose. My daughter Julia went into nursing school in order to learn to help others who were sick. She once wrote in an e-mail to a fellow student, "The only reason I keep my head above water is because I have a goal in life that I am determined to reach."

Jason Gaes, diagnosed with cancer as a child, responded by authoring *My Book for Kids with Cansur*—at age six! His purpose was to

> be a dr. who takes care of kids with cansur so when they say "Dr Jason, Sometimes I get so scared I'm going to die" or "you don't know how weird it is to be the only bald kid in your whole school" I can say "Oh yes I do. When I was a little boy I had cansur too. And look at all my hair now. Someday your hair will grow back too."

Purposes are often more aspirational than practical—goals that may never be achieved, like Don Quixote's "Impossible Dream." Yet as I consider the aforementioned purposes, it strikes me that their "degree of difficulty" is far less important than the passions they feed. Farmer Gary Lamb may never fully *alleviate world hunger,* but you get the sense that he truly believes in this purpose and lives a better life because of it. Jason Gaes didn't become a doctor (he became a golf pro!), but you can feel the passion in his purpose—and I'd bet that this helped him survive his cancer.

In a larger, spiritual sense, this passion is created by unlocking the "inner daimon" discussed in the previous chapter. This might feel like a tall order to many who wonder how to find and pursue a stronger purpose in their lives. So, to reduce the concept of purpose to its simplest elements, I suggest thinking of it as a higher-order *goal* that has deep *value*.

PURPOSE AS A GOAL

We have many big goals in our lives—getting into a good college, traveling to a particular destination, saving a certain sum for retirement—but also smaller day-to-day goals, such as mowing the lawn or getting milk for tomorrow's breakfast.

Researchers have known for years that setting a goal, regardless of its size, brings about more behavior change, motivation, effort, concentration, and persistence than does simply being asked to "do your best."[3] For example, I could probably get you to hold your breath significantly longer if I put in front of you a timer set for a specific period of time than if I were simply to ask you to hold it as long as you can.

An amazing thing about setting goals is that the higher you set them, the better you perform. Say you want to build your upper body and can do about fifteen push-ups at a time. Set a goal of ten push-ups and you can click them right off. Twenty might be a stretch, but you can just make it. How about thirty? So you try thirty and get to, well, twenty-four—which was super difficult, but you went well beyond what you thought was your limit.

A purpose in life can be not just difficult, but actually unattainable. In fact, mine is. I don't ever expect to announce, "Mission accomplished! I'm going to Disney World." Won't happen. I don't expect to help *everyone in the world* create a purpose in their lives, or to teach *every* student as if they were my own daughter. I'd like to, but it's probably beyond my grasp. Nonetheless my aspirational, unattainable purpose in life keeps me very engaged.

So let your purpose be big, lofty, even outrageous! I want to wake up in the morning with my purpose foremost in mind and go to bed at night knowing that I worked toward it. Did I help others create purpose in *their* lives? Did I spend enough quality time with my students? With my wife? Did I take time to enjoy my walk to work? If not, I've got some explaining to do—to myself.

DIFFERENT GOALS FOR DIFFERENT ROLES

Life is complicated. Goals don't have to be. In fact, researchers who study human performance have found that complex goals are easier to achieve if they're broken down into simpler ones. Watching an Olympic diver doing a backflip off a diving board will likely not help you do a better backflip. However, breaking down the complex acts into simple ones may keep you from doing a belly flop.

Breaking your life into the specific *roles* you have might help you compose a life purpose: Do you have a family purpose? A community purpose? A purpose in your work? Here's mine again: "To help others create a purpose in their lives, to teach every student as if they were my own daughter, to be an engaged husband and father, and to enjoy love and beauty."

I made a point of including community, work, family, and—why not?—my own personal purpose ("enjoy love and beauty"). This summarizes my overall purpose in life, and each component presents a goal that motivates me every day.

It also, alas, presents very real conflicts. For example, my work requires a lot of time with students—which can take time away from my family. Staying involved in my community can conflict with my work. And so on. If I catch myself spending too much time on one aspect of my purpose (for example, work) to the detriment of another aspect (for example, family), I ask myself whether this is really what I want to be doing. If not, why am I doing it?

A purpose, like a goal, also helps you focus on what's important and question what's not. For example, being a frequent traveler, a few years ago I found myself becoming obsessed with my frequent flyer miles. I was flying to Asia so often that I started dreaming up new classes of frequent flyer status:

Dear Dr. Strecher,
We are pleased to inform you that you've now reached Quantum Palladium Status and have the complete run of the plane. You may drink all of the drinks in the beverage cart, eat all the peanuts, fly the plane, play disco through the PA system, and dance with any of the flight attendants!
Sincerely,
The New Vic Strecher Airlines

But I started to wonder if I really wanted my headstone to read,

Vic Strecher

1955–2016

Three Trillion Frequent Flyer Miles

"I didn't know I had a peanut allergy!"

THE HEADSTONE TEST

When you find yourself conflicted between competing purposes, you might ask yourself, "Do I want [insert current obsession here] to be on my headstone?" Do you want to be the richest person in the graveyard? The most attractive person in the graveyard?

Twenty years ago Jerry Hirsch was developing shopping malls in Arizona as if he were popping corn. He made piles of money and seemed to have everything he wanted . . . until his wife left him. He sank into a severe depression and was even hospitalized. That's when he discovered Viktor Frankl's book, *Man's Search for Meaning.*

"It completely changed my life," Jerry says. "I started wondering what would be on my headstone, and realized it would be the number of Kmarts I built!" He quit what he was doing and founded the Lodestar Foundation, which leverages philanthropic impact through volunteerism and collaboration among nonprofit organizations. One of Lodestar's philosophical tenets is, "Happiness can only be found by identifying and striving to achieve a meaningful purpose for one's existence." In 2010, Barron's named Jerry one of the "25 Most Impactful Philanthropists."

"I don't do this for others," Jerry told me over lunch at an old Philadelphia diner. "I do it for *me*! I know that when I help others, I'm happy." This enlightened self-interest seems to have kept his depression at bay. He'd recently climbed Mount Kilimanjaro—in his seventies. As I wolfed down my meat loaf, I noticed the leafy, green salad he was tucking into. "I eat really healthy," he said in his clipped New York accent. "I hate the food but it keeps me alive longer. I have a lot more to do before I die."

PURPOSE AS A VALUE

Working toward goals—putting "points up on the board"—is fun and motivating. But without a deeper value, goals quickly become hollow. To create a motivating purpose in life, we must each ask ourselves, *What matters to me? What do I value?* In the previous chapter we discussed how these questions are central to Aristotle's approach to wellbeing. Also recall his emphasis on human agency—in being able to *choose* what we value.

If we could travel through history, we'd probably be struck by how little choice most people had in their lives. Kings, queens, pharaohs, popes, and khans all imposed a code of values from which they built their purposes—codes that generally took the form, "To serve [fill in the potentate] or face [fill in the banishment, imprisonment, or torture]." In modern times, we're still influenced by cultural norms of the past—we continue to borrow from that expired credit card—but given the choices we have in our society, many believe that we need to create our *own* values.

It's a little like cooking. Some of us follow recipes from a cookbook full of time-tested, traditional meals. Others make up their own recipes and cook from scratch. In my experience, the second group can be subdivided into two further categories: those who are good cooks to begin with, and those who should stay out of the kitchen.

Perhaps the most famous advocate of creating values from scratch was the philosopher Friedrich Nietzsche. In proclaiming that "God is dead!" Nietzsche was telling us to throw out our cookbooks. He begins *Thus Spoke Zarathustra* with an allegory of a camel who seeks to understand the world. Once the camel has sufficient education and knowledge of the world (has learned to cook), he transforms into a lion (becomes a really good cook). The lion, in turn, finds and destroys a dragon who has etched on every scale the words *thou shalt*. Once the dragon is defeated (the cookbooks are thrown away), the lion transforms into a child: innocent, untainted by societal norms (or meat loaf).

If you ever saw Stanley Kubrick's movie *2001: A Space Odyssey,* you'll recall the star child emerging at the end of the movie. I left the theater scratching my twelve-year-old head, but now I understand that his creature is in fact the child in Nietzsche's allegory. The story also inspired Richard Strauss's *Also sprach Zarathustra* (the same music playing as the star child appears). Nietzsche's influence on Kubrick is apparent in an interview conducted the same year as *2001: A Space Odyssey* was released: "The most terrifying fact about the universe is not that it is hostile but that it is indifferent, but if we can come to terms with this indifference, then our existence as a species can have genuine meaning. However vast the darkness, we must supply our own light."[4]

In 2014 I was invited to a symposium in a fifteenth-century monastery in a remote forest in Germany to speak about purpose in life, as part of a collaboration between the University of Heidelberg and the city of Mannheim. The symposium's theme was to "create a healthier Mannheim." As I was going through the benefits of having a purpose and some ideas for nurturing greater purpose, one of the participants raised his hand and said, "Well, Dr. Strecher, we know that Hitler had a purpose."

This wasn't an abstract comment. After all, I was in Germany—a country that threw its powerful collective purpose behind one man to create possibly the greatest suffering in world history.* The participant was asking a question fundamental to purpose: Do we accept *anyone's* chosen purpose? Are all values okay? If not, which are good and which are not, and who's to decide?

Let's respond to these questions with an initial warning: Philosophy, like cooking, can be a dangerous thing. A bad purpose can go horribly wrong. HANDLE WITH CARE! So how, exactly, do we handle our purpose with care? This is where Aristotle, again, helps

---

* Hitler was apparently a fan of Nietzsche—you can find a photo of Hitler staring reverently at a statue of the philosopher—so many assume that Nietzsche was a proto-Nazi. Nothing could be further from the truth. Nietzsche's Übermensch (superman) obviously appealed to Hitler's vision of a German master race, but Nietzsche was, in his own words, "anti-anti-Semitic." He was, in fact, a popular referent in the early twentieth-century Zionist movement.

us out, giving us buoys to guide our boat. What are the virtues we should value most deeply? His answer: courage, temperance, generosity, magnificence, justice, ambition, good temper, truthfulness, wittiness, friendliness, and modesty.

"Magnificence"? Okay, this may have been relevant for his top student, Alexander the Great, but it might seem odd to announce in modern times that you want to be magnificent. (Awesome, maybe?)

Benjamin Franklin, at the ripe old age of twenty, created his own list. It included temperance, silence, order, resolution, frugality, industry, sincerity, justice, moderation, cleanliness, tranquility, chastity, and humility. Franklin tracked his alignment (and famous *mis*-alignments) with these values every day until his death at eighty-four. They became the basis of what the sociologist Max Weber called the "protestant ethic," as well as of modern capitalism.[5] You can see how important it is to select one's values carefully!

Getting back to cooking. To make up your own recipe for living, you need to be a really good cook. We see many people throwing together a purpose in their lives willy-nilly, before they understand much about the world. Some of them grew up in abject poverty and don't understand the world. Some grew up in gated communities and don't understand the world. Some became terrorists. Some became disastrous global leaders. A great purpose in life follows from values that reflect an understanding of the world. This is the essence of the camel in Nietzsche's allegory: we must learn about the world if we're to create our own purposes. Prior to that, use a cookbook.

But regardless of how much we've seen and the ideas we've been exposed to, we can't *really* throw away the cookbook. We're brought up in cultures that hold certain values, and we can't just remove them from our worldview. But we *can* try to *understand* the values we were brought up with, and through this understanding we may be able to contrast new ways of seeing the world from the one we grew up with.

Following the historical catalogues of virtues people care about the most, modern social scientists have created many lists of their own. The World Values Survey is a global research project that regularly studies people's values and beliefs.[6] In the latest version of the survey, over seventy thousand people from fifty-one countries were asked to rate the importance of the following values: independence, wealth, security, pleasure, giving to society, giving to others, success, adventure, conformity, the environment, and tradition.

The survey reveals large differences between countries. In China, for example, wealth and success are held in far more esteem than pleasure is; in the Netherlands, the opposite holds true. (Having lived in the Netherlands, and hanging out in pubs filled with massively drunk people painted orange, I can happily attest to this, hangover and all.) In the United States, the Netherlands, and China, "doing something for the good of society" is ranked first, whereas in Russia it comes in fifth.

There are gender differences, too. In the United States, men are more likely to rank independence, wealth, success, pleasure, and adventure highly, whereas women on average tend to rank security, society, the environment, and tradition more highly. Mars and Venus.*

---

* These tendencies, of course, are based only on averages. Many of the people in our lives (at least in mine) don't fit these averages at all.

Also, younger Americans are more likely to value independence, wealth, pleasure, and adventure.

Values are also clearly aligned with political leanings. The World Values Survey found that in the United States, conservatives tend to value wealth, security, conformity, and tradition, but liberals tend to place more value on the environment. Success is valued by both the political Right and Left, but primarily at the far *ends* of the spectrum. Liberals and conservatives both seem to value pleasure. (Apparently hedonism transcends political affiliation!)

Also as you might expect, wealthier people throughout the world are more likely to value wealth and success than are those less well off. However, one of the most important values across all countries and incomes is *helping others*.

This very brief summary illustrates that the country we grew up in, our gender, and whether we have a large or small bank account all influence the values we hold dear—and ultimately the purpose in life we create. There are clearly lots of other broad-brush factors that influence our values—our religious affiliation (if any), our race and ethnicity, our education, and many others—but you get the point: unless we were raised by wolves (who I guess have their own set of values), we've been imbued with a set of core values simply by virtue of growing up. It's hard to be the Nietzschean lion and throw away the cookbooks even if we want to!

But we also get our values from other people. Of course, our parents influence our values as we grow up, but as we become adults and more interested in a self-determined purpose, whom do we look to?

WHAT WOULD BOGIE DO?

Aristotle said that we obtain the virtues of a eudaimonic life from the emulation of worthy people. Emulation isn't so much trying to replicate another person's life (all too common in our modern world of wannabes and fanboys) as it is *utilizing the principles* of the person's life for self-improvement.[7] We may strive to emulate Humphrey Bogart's independence and toughness, but do we have to dress the way he did? Talk the way he did?

Dressing or talking like Bogie will not make us tougher or more independent; it only makes us look like a person who does not want to be him- or herself. The growth from imitation to emulation is exemplified to perfection in the Woody Allen comedy, *Play It Again, Sam.* Toward the end, Allan Felix (played by Allen) is talking to his role model, Humphrey Bogart (played by Jerry Lacy):

> **Bogart:** That was great. You've, uh, you've really developed yourself a little style.
>
> **Allan:** Yeah, I do have a certain amount of style, don't I?
>
> **Bogart:** Well, I guess you won't be needing me anymore. There's nothing I can tell you now that you don't already know.
>
> **Allan:** I guess that's so. I guess the secret's not being you; it's being me. True, you're . . . you're not too tall and kind of ugly, but . . . what the hell—I'm short enough and ugly enough to succeed on my own.
>
> **Bogart:** Humph. Here's looking at you, kid.

We all need people that we consider worthy to look up to and ask, "What would [worthy person] do?"

In 2003 I took my older daughter, Rachael, to South Africa. I was working for the National Cancer Institute on a project designed to help South African adolescents reduce their use of tobacco and other drugs. We were focusing most of our attention on three schools: a fancy, nearly all-white school; a mixed-race school; and one in a very poor township called Gugulethu.

Rachael, then sixteen, was the photo editor of her school's newspaper (she'd later become an Associated Press photographer in the Middle East). I thought she might aid my feeble attempts to communicate with adolescents. She did. Using a technique called "photovoice," Rachael handed disposable cameras to twenty-four teenagers with a simple request: for the next four days, shoot pictures of *what you value*.

I expected them to come back with photos of objects. I was wrong. They brought us pictures of people.

In Gugulethu, we rarely saw photos of the children's parents. That was because most of them were dead. AIDS had swept their parents' generation away in coffins stacked two and three high on top of cars. These children would hold up the pictures they took and say, "This is my coach; he's like my father. He tells me not to drink. Not to smoke." "This is my cousin. He tells me I'm too beautiful to smoke." "This is my brother. He tells me what I must do." "This is my neighbor. She acts like my mother."

Emulation. It happens everywhere. Visiting the homes (often corrugated metal boxes) of these teenagers, I met many of the subjects of those pictures—coaches, cousins, brothers, and neighbors. They were indeed worthy of emulation. Even in this seemingly hopeless environment, people sought out values to provide meaning to their lives. Those in Gugulethu who didn't have these people were lost. As one teen movingly put it, "I could not live my life without them."

I also noticed that as the students discussed the people they valued, they became less defensive. Expressing their values opened a door into their problems, their hopes, and their desire for a better life.

VALUES AFFIRMATION

People with a strong life purpose are more likely to live longer, healthier lives. Why? One reason may be that they engage in healthy behaviors and are more willing to change unhealthy behaviors. Why? The answer may be related to the values component of purpose.

When we're told that we need to change something in our lives—to become more physically active or quit smoking—we often go on the defensive:

"My heart has only so many beats in it. Why make it go faster?"

"Why, if you lined up end-to-end all the cigarettes my uncle smoked, they would go to the moon and back . . . and he was finally hit by a bus! He was ninety-eight, and even after he was dead they had to stomp on his lungs to make them stop!"

If we first ask a smoker to consider their purposeful, deeply held values, the smoker becomes less defensive and more willing to consider quitting. Over the past decade, there have been dozens of studies examining the impact of self-affirmation on reducing defensiveness to change. Affirming core values has been shown to reduce resistance to improving physical activity and diet, quitting smoking, and reducing alcohol consumption and excessive sun exposure, among other self-improving behaviors.

These findings are important to public health professionals, who often use fear-arousing messages in an attempt to break through defensiveness. Beyond health messages, consider the increasingly shrill screeds from our politicians and talk-show pundits. Scaring and yelling at people usually don't work—human beings are remarkably adept at defending their egos and build extensive mechanisms for doing so. The affirmation of purposeful values is a *positive* approach to behavior change. The Temperance Society and political polemicists may not approve, but by considering our values—this central component of purpose—we begin to find our inner self, unclouded by defensiveness.

IN SEARCH OF THE DAIMON INSIDE

In the previous chapter, I mentioned the golden figurines hidden inside ancient terra-cotta busts of Greek gods, meant to represent the daimon or inner self. Our research team grew interested in learning how the affirmation of core values works in the brain: whether values affirmation activates the "self" and whether this activation leads to behavior change.

Led by University of Pennsylvania researcher Emily Falk,[8] we started with an already-identified part of the brain related to the "self."[9] It's in an area called the ventromedial prefrontal cortex, affectionately known as the vmPFC. It's easy to find: Point to your forehead, right between your eyes or slightly higher. An inch or so in dwells the vmPFC. When people are processing information about the self, this part of the brain becomes active.

Next, we needed a behavior to study. We invited into the study a group of sedentary people who would benefit from physical activity and gave each of them an accelerometer to measure activity changes. After a week of learning about each participant's activity patterns, we put them into a magnetic resonance imager. While scanning their brains, we asked half of them to think about the values they cared about the *most*. For example, we'd ask a person who valued religion to "think of a time when religious values might give you a purpose in life." Participants in the control group were asked to think about the values they cared *least* about.

Then for four weeks following the scanning session, while still monitoring their physical activity, we sent all participants daily messages about increasing it. Participants in the values affirmation group also received messages about their most important values, whereas those in the control group received messages about their least important values.

The results strongly confirmed our initial hypotheses: compared to the control group, those in the group who considered their most important core values had greater activation of their vmPFC—the part of the brain related to the self—and went on to increase their physical activity over the next month. In fact, the more the vmPFC became activated, the more physical activity occurred over the next month. The affirmation of core purposeful values seems to "open our mind" to change.

But what does it mean to open our mind? What's happening to our "self" when we're thinking about important values? In a fascinating study entitled "Why Does Writing About Important Values Reduce Defensiveness?," psychologist Jennifer Crocker and her colleagues asked study participants either to write about their most important value and why it was meaningful to them (the values affirmation group) or to write about their least important value and why it might be important and meaningful to other people (the control group). Next, the subjects were asked to rate how the essay they wrote *made them feel*. Finally, they tested the participants' defensiveness. Subjects affirming their most important values felt *love, connectedness,* and *empathy,* and these *transcending feelings* reduced their defensiveness.

WHAT MATTERS MOST

The life purposes mentioned at the beginning of this chapter represent goals, but more importantly they're a product of deeply held values. The purposes of Samuel Barber and Dexter Gordon reflect the artistic values of creativity and free expression. For Gary Lamb and Harry Blackmun, they're the prosocial values of compassion and empathy. For Madeleine L'Engle, they're the spiritual values of living fully and in the moment.

Many people confuse or conflate "purpose" with "meaning" in life. There's a very important distinction. Meaning in life asks the question, "Why am I here?" As we'll discuss later, responses to this question vary greatly and may even include, "No reason." Purpose in life is concerned with what we most deeply value, and purposeful living is concerned with whether we're living for what matters most.

So what matters most to you? As we've discussed in this chapter, our values are a product of our cultural environment, our education, and our experience of the human condition. As we contemplate these values, we take the first step toward purposeful living.

FINDING YOUR PURPOSE

Here's a six-step guide that might help you discover your purpose in life:

Step 1: Consider what matters most to you. Here's a list of core values. From the list, select the three you care about the most in your life. If you have a value that's not on the list, go ahead and use that one.

- Achievement
- Community
- Creativity
- Enjoyment
- Expertise

- Independence
- Kindness
- Relationships
- Reputation
- Responsibility

- Security
- Self-Control
- Spirituality
- Tradition
- Vitality

Once you've selected your top three values, spend a little time thinking about, or better yet, writing about why each value is important to you. (This will begin activating your vmPFC—the part of your brain associated with the "self.")

Step 2: Think about a person or people you'd like to emulate (*not* imitate). Someone in your family? A historical figure? A public figure? A cartoon character? This is *your* purpose and you can choose whatever mix of people you like. However, whether it's your aunt Sue, Amelia Earhart, Humphrey Bogart, or Bugs Bunny, just remember, to paraphrase Kurt Vonnegut, you are who you choose to be, so be careful who you choose to be.

Step 3: Take the headstone test. That's right—draw a headstone, write your name on it, write in your date of birth. For the date of death, write "TODAY." What would your epitaph be? What would you want people to say about you at your memorial service?

Step 4: Now that you've primed the pump and are a bit more in touch with your inner daimon, ask yourself, "What are the goals in my life that matter the most?" To make this easier, you might want to break these into personal, family, work (or school), and community goals that you deeply value. For ideas, you might want to go to the beginning of this chapter and read through the purposes of others (notice that they all begin with "To . . .").

Step 5: Assemble these valued goals into an overall life purpose. This is where you want to stop and ask yourself, "Is this purpose bigger than myself?" Ask yourself this simple, timeless question: "In living toward this purpose, will I treat others the way I would like to be treated?" Make sure the suit fits.

Step 6: Wear the suit. Post your purpose in a place you'll see every day. Make sure you can recite your purpose to yourself or others. Consider sharing your purpose with the people who are close to you. If the purpose doesn't fit, change it until it does.

You now possess the most important statement of your life. It defines who you are. I've collected thousands of purposes in my work. So far, no two have been the same. It's your fingerprint. Your DNA. It's the statement that separates you from your boss, the street urchin in Mumbai, and your jerk of a brother-in-law. Your "best purpose" becomes your inner motivator, turning on the ignition switch in your brain to transcend the noise in your life and focus on what matters most.

4

SELF-TRANSCENDENCE

Only to the extent that someone is living out this self-transcendence of human existence is he truly human or does he become his true self. He becomes so, not by concerning himself with his self's actualization, but by forgetting himself and giving himself, overlooking himself and focusing outward.

VIKTOR FRANKL[1]

Make the other band members look and sound
good. Bring out the best in them; that's your job.

CHRISSIE HYNDE[2]

AT ROUGHLY 2,200 MILES, THE APPALACHIAN TRAIL EXTENDS FROM
Georgia to Maine. To hike the entire trail, most people start in early
spring and finish in late summer or early fall—a stretch of about five
to seven months. This works out to about twelve miles a day, every
day—a significant amount of hiking. It's been estimated that fewer
than one in five hikers complete their journey. The terrain, illness,
injuries, and weather extremes make the hike a life challenge.

Apparently no one told Jennifer Pharr Davis about the time it
should take to hike the Appalachian Trail.[3] Or if they did, she didn't
listen. Pharr Davis wanted to break the speed record for hiking the
trail. To do so, she would need to average *forty-five miles a day for
forty-six days*.

Despite extensive preparation, however, Pharr Davis broke down just twelve days into her hike. Severe shin splints and four straight days of diarrhea drained her body of energy. She recounts, "I was already way off pace, and thought 'there is no way I can get the record.' I gave up."

Upon reaching the next checkpoint, she told her husband, Brew, that she was quitting. "Brew was not OK with it." Looking into his eyes, she came to a life-changing realization, "Until then, everything had been about *me* and the record. I was a slave to the record, it was all I was thinking about."

The realization sparked a major shift in her purpose. "I just totally released from the record. I started hiking out of a greater faith. I wanted to honor my God, to get back to the reasons that got me hooked on hiking to begin with—a love for the wilderness, a love for my husband, and to use my gift. I remembered that I feel closest to God when I am hiking up and down the trail as a part of nature, when I am loving my husband, when I am relishing in my gift. All of a sudden, the hike was no longer about a record, it was no longer about me. The whole thing became an act of worship to something greater than myself."

For the next thirty-four days Jennifer Pharr Davis averaged over *forty-seven miles per day,* shattering the record by twenty-six hours.

SOMETHING GREATER THAN YOURSELF

Jennifer Pharr Davis shifted her perspective from self-enhancing to self-transcending—and improved her performance. You may have heard of Abraham Maslow's hierarchy of needs. For most of his career, Abraham Maslow, the founder of humanistic psychology, viewed self-actualization as the pinnacle of human existence—the ultimate stage of development, only reachable after other more basic needs, such as physical or safety needs, have been met. This emphasis on an individual's own actualization heralded the "me generation"—baby boomers intent on jogging, dieting, and meditating (or navel-gazing, in the words of their detractors) to reach "*self*-realization" and "*self*-fulfillment."

Viktor Frankl thought that this self-focus was narcissistic and ultimately detrimental to the self. He suggested that real fulfillment in life occurs only when a person transcends the self. In the latter part of his career, Maslow understood the importance of Frankl's words, writing in 1969, "The fully developed (and very fortunate) human being working under the best conditions tends to be motivated by values which transcend his *self*. They are not selfish anymore in the old sense of that term."[4]

Maslow began to study "transcenders," finding that these individuals were better able to see connections between disparate ideas, making them better innovators and discoverers. Transcending scientists, he discovered, exhibited "humility, a sense of ignorance, a feeling of smallness, awe before the tremendousness of the universe."[5] I find it remarkable that Abraham Maslow, at the pinnacle of his field, would change his hugely popular model, saying essentially, "I was wrong." Who does that?

Going into her hike, Jennifer Pharr Davis knew the "how" of

her endeavor. She had the right knowledge and the right training. She even had a "why"—but it wasn't the right "why." Pharr Davis broke the hiking record because she finally understood her transcending purpose for hiking.

Coaches and teachers are usually able to provide the knowledge and skills to perform, but the great coaches and teachers help to find the right why in their protégés. In doing so, they teach wisdom.

TRANSCENDENT COACHES

"What you are as a person is far more important than what you are as a basketball player," said legendary UCLA Bruins basketball coach John Wooden.[6] You may be thinking, "That's easy to say when you have Kareem Abdul-Jabbar in your starting lineup." But one could argue that great players went to these great coaches because they sought wisdom, not just trophies.

As Abdul-Jabbar said about his former coach, "He wanted to win, but not more than anything . . . My relationship with him has been one of the most significant of my life . . . The consummate teacher, he taught us that the best you are capable of is victory enough, and that you can't walk until you crawl, that gentle but profound truth about growing up."[7]

Can a coach transcend winning? There's little doubt that great coaches are highly competitive and committed to winning, but I've never quite been comfortable with Red Sanders's quote, "Winning isn't everything; it's the only thing."[8] I believe that the greatest coaches care more about the *wisdom derived from the process that led to winning* than the winning itself.

Can you remember who won last year's Super Bowl? I can't. And I don't really care. I *do* care about the wisdom gleaned from watching the coordination of effort, concentration, and persistence when combined with a purpose; there's wisdom in this orchestration that transcends the sport. Winning is not everything *or* the only thing. As Dean Smith, among the winningest coaches in college basketball history, said, "If you make every game a life-and-death thing, you're going to have problems. You'll be dead a lot."[9]

TRANSCENDENT TEACHERS

A student recently asked me for advice to overcome his difficulties in calculus, which he found both hard and excruciatingly boring. I had trouble coming up with an answer, as I thought of Euclid's response over 2,500 years ago to his king's request to provide an easier way to learn math: "There is no royal road to geometry." Learning the details of mathematics or a "hard science" can be boring and is, well . . . hard.

You may not be able to make math more enjoyable, but you can make it more bearable. In a recent study with the great title *Boring but Important: A Self-Transcendent Purpose for Learning Fosters Academic Self-Regulation,*[10] David Yeager and his colleagues tested whether an intervention designed to enhance a self-transcendent purpose for learning could improve GPA in STEM courses (science, technology, engineering, and mathematics). They gave one group of ninth graders a thirty-minute web-based intervention designed to promote a self-transcending purpose. The carefully thought-out program is itself worth describing.

At the beginning of a grading quarter, researchers asked the students to write about social injustices that they found particularly troublesome. "Sometimes the world isn't fair . . . What are some ways that you think the world could be a better place?" The intervention then provided a normative message to the students: that "many students like you" were motivated to learn "so they can make a positive contribution to the world." Finally, students in this group were asked to write a testimonial to future students about their purpose for learning. Some of the testimonials included,

> "I would like to get a job as some sort of genetic researcher. I would use this job to help improve the world by possibly engineering crops to produce more food, or something like that."

> "I believe learning in school will give me the rudimentary skills to survive in the world. Science will give me a good base for my career in environmental engineering. I want to be able to solve our energy problems."

Compared with ninth graders who received a control exercise, the students receiving the purpose intervention had significantly higher grades in STEM courses by the end of the grading quarter.

Even more remarkably, students with lower initial grade point averages responded *most* positively to the intervention.

Should teachers help their students to transcend their focus beyond simply getting a good grade? Numerous research studies and my own teaching experience say yes. In fact, the more students focus solely on their grade, the less well they perform. I see students becoming engaged, and performing better, in school when they're trying to master the course material with a purpose in mind.

We don't typically see teachers of STEM courses discuss how the mastery of a subject leads to solving larger social issues, but what if this discussion became the starting point of learning these hard subjects? What if the relevance was built directly into the instruction?

TRANSCENDENT VERSUS SELFISH

It's commonly believed that people are naturally selfish and need to be *taught*—by parents, schools, churches—to become transcending, altruistic, and empathic. Indeed, if our true nature is to be selfish, then wouldn't this "I've got mine, Jack" approach to living make sense? From an evolutionary perspective, don't people benefit most from being selfish? Or to reverse the question, if self-transcendence is part of the nature of living things, why don't animals act this way?

As a matter of fact, they do. The biologist Frans de Waal, who studies altruistic behavior among dolphins, whales, elephants, chimpanzees, and bonobos, concludes that "there is now increasing evidence that the brain is hardwired for social connection, and that the same empathy mechanism proposed to underlie human altruism may underlie the directed altruism of other animals."[11]

Dolphins, whales, and elephants are majestic creatures. But when we think of empathic behavior, the *rat* probably doesn't come to mind. Maybe it should. In an important recent study,[12] researchers started by placing a rat in a cage. A second rat was further confined within a smaller clear cage inside the larger one. After a bit of training, the first rat was able to free the second, which the rat did almost every time. Interestingly, the first rat did the same thing *even* when a container of chocolate chips (which rats love) was placed in the outer cage! It would first free the caged rat and they would *share* the chocolate chips. Apparently transcendent behavior transcends the human race.

Do we really need to train children to become transcending? It turns out that scientists observe altruistic behavior in infants even before such values can be consciously learned. Research on babies as young as fourteen months find naturally occurring altruistic behavior—babies helping each other fetch out-of-reach objects or opening cabinets. They do this without any rewards from adults. In fact, external rewards from adults can actually *undermine* the behavior.[13]

Studies showing that we're hardwired to be empathic and altruistic run counter to many Western religious perspectives. I was taught in Sunday school that we were born with "original sin" and that religion was organized to put us on the straight-and-narrow road to being a good person.

I was recently with a Hindu priest in one of the most beautiful, peaceful places in the world: Bali. When I told him about my Sunday school education, the priest laughed out loud. "In our philosophy you are born with the *atman*, the true self. It's the exposure to the world that makes us sinful." (By the way, the "atman" sounds a bit like Aristotle's "daimon," doesn't it?) I've heard countless parents say, "We're not that religious but we take our children to church so they'll learn right from wrong." If children are, as these studies suggest, born with the *right* in them, isn't it our responsibility to let these virtues flourish?

Is there a downside to purely altruistic behavior? In his book *Give and Take*,[14] University of Pennsylvania psychologist Adam Grant points out that purely selfless giving has significant costs, such as being a chump that's always taken advantage of, and is not healthy in the long run.

Grant talks about being "otherish"—helpful and altruistic while preserving your own goals—to create a win-win situation. My work purpose—"to teach every student as if they were my own daughter"—can get me into trouble. As word about this purpose spreads through my classes, I get dozens of students each week who want to speak with me. If I'm not careful and "otherish," my family, work, and person purposes start suffering. I therefore need to set limits and find strategies for supporting students while not necessarily filling my days with meetings.

Beyond setting limits, however, is creating connections between purposes. A family who volunteers together in the community may be connecting two purposes. Many people connect their personal and community purposes with their work purpose.

TRANSCENDENT BUSINESSES

Near the British Museum in London is the headquarters of Bupa, one of the largest health-care companies in the world. I was there to meet with their chief executive officer, Stuart Fletcher. I'd learned ahead of time that Fletcher had a tradition of placing each of his senior leaders beneath a blinding spotlight and asking them what their purpose was. The ordeal reminded me of George Bernard Shaw's suggestion that we should all "appear before a board every five years, and justify our existence . . . on pain of liquidation." What, I wondered as I waited in his anteroom, does Stuart Fletcher do with employees who are unable to define their purpose? Is a trapdoor involved?

Entering his CEO-ish office I encountered an ebullient man with bright eyes and a bounce in his step. In fact, he reminded me of Tigger from Winnie the Pooh—counter to my stereotype of a world-class CEO. In fact, he didn't fit any stereotype.

Our conversation began by discussing the purpose of Bupa, which was displayed prominently throughout the headquarters: "*longer, healthier, happier lives*." It was clearly more than just a slogan dreamed up by the marketing department. Not only does this purpose provide an ethical compass in the everyday decisions Fletcher and his people make, it also motivates his personal behavior to take the stairs and walk many miles a week.

I asked him where his interest in purpose came from. He responded slowly, eyes welling up: "I don't generally talk about this, but when I was a child, my elder brother was killed in an accident. It shattered my parents, and for me, his death taught me that we're not here forever—life is very precious. In the brief time that we are here, the possibility is to make it really count!"

The ubiquitous corporate mission, "To make the world a better place," has practically become a joke. We know better, and as many business-focused people (the more candid ones, anyway) have told me, "The ultimate goal of any business is to maximize shareholder value." What about the "make the world a better place"? What about the customer? The employees? The community? Do they matter?

To Ari Weinzweig, it matters. Ari, cofounder of Zingerman's Deli, Roadhouse, Bakehouse, and other businesses in Ann Arbor, Michigan, started a deli with his partner, Paul Saginaw, in a tiny space in an unpopular part of town. They now oversee more than $50 million of business a year.

Ari calls himself a "lapsed anarchist."[15] Anarchy, he explained over a cup of tea, is unfortunately typified by a bunch of bomb-tossing Bolsheviks. But the word simply means "without hierarchy," and Ari's approach to running the Zingerman's businesses perfectly exemplifies this counterintuitive approach. For one, his budget meetings are open to any Zingerman's employee. You can find Ari at the meetings—sitting on the side or in back. Others run the meeting, pointing out successes, problems, and solutions. Anyone—from the managers to the dishwashers—can, and does, come up with solutions.

People in Ann Arbor love Zingerman's: the customers, the employees, and the community. It's also famous internationally. Among many other accolades, it's been named "the coolest small com-

pany in America" by *Inc.* magazine. Ari and Paul even gave the com-
mencement address to the University of Michigan's class of 2015. Yet,
if you go to Zingerman's Roadhouse for dinner, you'll likely see Ari in
his black T-shirt and jeans, gliding from table to table to refill water
glasses and offer extra barbecue sauce for their Roadhouse Ribs.

The company's mission statement says it all:

> We share the Zingerman's Experience
> Selling food that makes you happy
> Giving service that makes you smile
> In passionate pursuit of our mission
> Showing love and care in all our actions
> To enrich as many lives as we possibly can.

Ari says that this mission is the foundation of their business. "No
matter how lost or frustrated we may feel, our mission is always there,
much like the North Star, to help guide us." I've spoken with business people who've said, "Well, it's easy to act this way when you're
a $50 million company." Let's not reverse cause and effect here. Ari
and Paul *started* their business this way and became successful, just as
transcending coaches *started* this way and became successful, just as
transcending people *started* this way and became successful.

In a book entitled *Firms of Endearment,*[16] business school profes-
sors Raj Sisodia, David Wolfe, and Jag Sheth identified twenty-eight
companies based on the strength of, and demonstrated dedication to,
a revenue-transcending purpose. You've heard of many of these companies: REI, Trader Joe's, 3M, Costco. They're loved by their custom-

ers, employees, and surrounding communities. They were deliberately *not* selected for this study because of their financial performance, but because of their purpose.

Sisodia and his colleagues matched the financial performance from 1998 to 2013 of their twenty-eight Firms of Endearment against the Standard & Poor's 500 and companies selected from the *Good to Great* book by Jim Collins.[17] (Good to Great companies were selected based on their managerial and financial acumen; dedication to a transcending purpose was not one of the criteria. The tobacco giant Philip Morris, for example, is on the Good to Great company list.)

Three years into the comparison, the Good to Great companies were returning over 200 percent of investment, more than doubling the performance of both the Firms of Endearment and the S&P 500. It looked at that time like the focus on revenue, regardless of purpose, resulted in more revenue.

By 2013, over the fifteen-year period, the Good to Great companies returned 263 percent of investment, completely swamping the 118 percent return from the S&P 500. But hold on to your stock portfolio: by 2013, *the Firms of Endearment ended up returning 1,681 percent of investment!*

The lesson from this study? I believe it's the same lesson we can learn from purpose among individuals: that a transcending purpose results in a greater return. It's also more fun.

In his famous book *Working,*[18] Studs Terkel said that work "is about the search, too, for daily meaning as well as daily bread, for recognition as well as for cash, for astonishment rather than torpor;

in short, for a sort of life rather than a Monday through Friday sort of dying." Yet torpor and dying is the situation that the employees of most businesses find themselves in.

A 2013 Gallup study[19] of American employees found that those engaged in their work had 37 percent lower absenteeism than unengaged employees. Unfortunately, they also found that seven in ten workers are "not engaged" or "actively disengaged" in their work and that these workers were far more likely to have chronic health problems. The study found that the number one way to minimize disengagement is to focus on the organization's purpose.

Pointing out to employees that their actions affect others can result in transcending behaviors—and save lives. In an elegant study,[20] Adam Grant and his colleague David Hofmann compared the effectiveness of two different posted signs in encouraging handwashing by health-care professionals in hospitals. They found that a sign that emphasized the self-transcending purpose of patient safety ("Hand hygiene prevents patients from catching diseases") resulted in 45 percent more sanitizing soap gel used, whereas a self-only purpose sign ("Hand hygiene prevents you from catching diseases") resulted in 4 percent *less* soap gel used!

DIRTY JOBS

But what if you're working in a tedious, low-paying, low-status job? How can you possibly find "daily meaning as well as daily bread"? There is an old story of two bricklayers asked why they do their job. One says, "Well, I get a penny a brick." The other says, "I'm making a cathedral." Jane Dutton, a professor in the University of Michigan's business school, studies the difference between working for a buck and what she calls "job crafting."

Jane and her colleagues[21] once interviewed custodians at the University of Michigan Health System and found that many were, indeed, simply working for money. Others, however, crafted their jobs into something more transcending. "I'm a part of the medical team," said one custodian. "I put a fresh flower in front of a patient who's in a coma. If she ever wakes up, the first thing she'll see is something beautiful." My daughter Julia spent a lot of time in the hospital, and once in a while we'd see a custodian reading a book to one of the patients whose parents never had time to visit.

The researchers asked the custodians what the hardest part of their job was. They all said it was waxing the floors—a tough job involving first stripping the old wax, then replacing it with fresh wax that needed to dry. Walking on wet wax would ruin the job and the custodian would need to redo the entire process. That's why they put up signs reading "Fresh wax. Do not walk here."

They then asked whether anyone walked on the wax. "The doctors" was a common reply. "And when they walked on the wet floor," said one custodian, "it was like they were walking all over me." An organization that's successful in getting its employees—even employees with jobs that generally suck—aligned with its purpose can increase their productivity, reduce absenteeism, and increase engagement in their work. At minimum, their jobs should suck less.

Large corporations often have mission workshops requiring all new employees to learn a treacly mission statement and watch an inspirational video or two with cloying music à la the illegitimate spawn of Kenny G and John Tesh. A human resource representative then asks employees to describe how the mission relates to their life. Kill me now.

As with individuals, an organizational purpose must be authentic and must be lived daily as a dynamic process. As the "firms of endearment" found at an organizational level, and Jane Dutton and her colleagues found with hospital custodians, a work purpose can create greater revenue *and* greater job satisfaction: a win-win.

TRANSCENDENT YOU

Equating the foregoing with your own life, here's a little test to give yourself: Are your conversations with others spent describing your prostate-specific antigen (PSA) level or your cholesterol numbers? Do you spend a lot of time complaining about rude waitresses and inattentive sales persons, or that one relative or coworker who's always dissing you? George Bernard Shaw said, "This is the true joy in life, the being used for a purpose recognized by yourself as a mighty one . . . the being a force of Nature instead of a feverish selfish little clod of ailments and grievances."[22]

It's so easy spending our lives complaining and blaming others. People often eventually quit complaining and find a true joy in life—

when they're dying. A recent study[23] of people going through palliative care before death recorded the following transcending statements about the final stage of their lives:

"I think that this is probably, truthfully, the best time of my life. Because I see so clearly. Everything is so magnified, clarified. And I think that there is something, there is a lot that people forget in the mundane, in the simplicity of life. The simplicity. Simple. Simple. Elegant. Beautiful."

"It's like you're in this envelope of just pure love and contentment. And I walk in that every day. I wake up grateful. I go to bed grateful. I laugh a lot. You know you live in the real world but you don't have to always live in that reality. You can rise above that."

"And, that thing I could say was learning about love and learning about the importance of giving . . . *because this is not a way that I used to be*" (emphasis mine).

For this last person, it took dying to begin living. For others, as with Aristotle and Socrates, it took examination and reason.

For me, it took a miracle.

5

MIRACLES, GOD, AND THE AFTERLIFE

The thing is to find a truth which is true for me,

to find the idea for which I can live and die.

SØREN KIERKEGAARD[1]

SEPTEMBER 1, 2000

Looking up at the medicines dripping into her thin, bruised arms, I asked my daughter, "Okay, Julia, what's the roman numeral for four?" Her tired eyes narrowed a little in thought; moments later she wrote "IV" on her paper. "Good job!"

That was the job of my wife, Jeri, and me—to keep Julia thinking, to keep her occupied with anything other than the hospital, her condition, and the suffering of the children around her. "Let's do some more—you're really getting it." But she was clearly too tired, and the drugs she was taking had given her a bad headache.

"Does she really need to learn roman numerals for homework?" I wondered. I'd never used them myself. For that matter, would she need *anything* we were teaching her? Julia was nine and waiting for a second heart transplant. The first heart she'd received, eight years earlier, was wearing out. We'd spent most of the summer in the hospital with her. We didn't tell her about the boy down the hall who had just died after his transplant.

SEPTEMBER 6, 2000

Julia's condition was worsening. Her heart was beating irregularly. She'd had a seizure the night before and was moved into a new unit. I said good night to her, and a nurse found an empty bed down the hall for me, but I couldn't sleep. I stayed up until 1:30 A.M. watching the U.S. Open tennis tournament. Todd Martin versus Carlos Moya. Martin was down two sets to nothing, and though he looked as sick and exhausted as many of the patients in the hospital, he somehow willed himself to a victory over Moya in the fifth set. From this moving display of resilience, I thought to myself, "Maybe Julia has it in her, too," and fell asleep.

I was shaken awake at 4:00 A.M. by a nurse, who told me with tears in her eyes, "Julia's heart has stopped twice in the last half hour. They're still working on her, but it doesn't look good." I got my clothes on and walked with the nurse to the intensive care unit (ICU). They wouldn't let me in to see her, but they helped me call my wife. I couldn't speak to her—my throat was completely shut.

When Jeri arrived, we waited silently for another hour in a private room. The doctors finally came in, sat down, and told us that Julia's heart had stopped beating on its own six times over the past two and a half hours, sometimes for as long as fifteen minutes. After a series of tests, the neurologist found that Julia was completely unresponsive to light or any stimulus and was probably severely or completely mentally impaired. Her organs were beginning to fail, and they were quite certain that she wouldn't make it through another arrest. With our consent, a "do not resuscitate" order was placed at her bedside.

When we were finally brought in to see our daughter, Jeri said, "She's gone. She's not in there." I agreed. Julia's dilated eyes were wide open, staring at nothing. Only the respirator kept her chest moving. Her skin was blue, and there were still tubes running in and out of her iodine-stained body. She had large burn marks from the defibrillation paddles used to continually restart her heart.

A curtain was closed around us, and we whispered good-bye to our daughter.

When we returned to the doctors, Jeri had the self-transcending presence of mind to ask whether Julia's organs could be donated to others in need. The doctors agreed that some of her organs might still be useful and sent for a "harvest team" to fly in and make a final evaluation. The process would take hours and, nearly suffocating in the hospital, I suggested that Jeri and I, along with our daughter Rachael, now fourteen, go for a walk. In the adjacent park we talked about Julia and about our new life as a trio rather than a quartet. We would still play music. We'd still be a family. I looked up into the bright blue sky and said that it was a pretty day to go to heaven. We tried to take turns sobbing; somebody had to keep it together enough to keep the tissues coming.

Although her death wasn't official—a certificate hadn't been prepared or signed—word that Julia had died leaked out of the hospital that morning to her elementary school, which promptly called in social workers who broke the news to her young classmates. Meanwhile, walking back to the hospital, we decided to see Julia one last time. They'd kept the curtain closed around her in the ICU. The doctors had removed most of the tubes and cleaned her body.

But . . .

. . . *she was moving.* Her head was bobbing spastically up and down; her tongue was sticking in and out. Her eyes were still wide open, yet she was clearly blind. Her arm was lurching out at an odd angle. The attending doctor suggested that these movements could be the result of low-level brain activity—a kinder term for "death throes." It certainly didn't look like deliberate or organized movement. In fact, the spastic motions scared me—it looked like she was suffering. For God's sake, how long did this have to go on?

Then, out of the blue, Jeri asked, "Julia, do you have to go potty?" Spastically, Julia's head nodded. Jeri's eyes locked with mine. Slipping my finger into Julia's hand, I whispered into her ear, "If you can hear me, squeeze my hand." I felt a slight squeeze. At least I thought I did.

I turned to the doctor. I realized that even if she made it through these heart attacks, if she was mentally impaired, she'd be dropped from the transplant list, just to suffer a lingering death. A demonstration of genuine mental acuity would be required. But how? She was blind. Her responses up to that point could have been those of a two-year-old. But she could hear . . . maybe.

I had a thought. "Remember, Julia, when we learned roman numerals last week? Can you squeeze my hand IV times?"

I felt four very deliberate squeezes.

Within two minutes a team was working frantically to get Julia's organs functioning again. Three days later, she could see. In fact, she was playing Bach on an electronic piano at her bedside in the ICU. A doctor walked into her room and cried. Another doctor told us that she'd never practice medicine in the same way again. And another two days later, Julia got a new heart.

After a few months, Julia's fourth-grade teacher half kiddingly asked us whether the donor of Julia's new heart was exceptional in math. "I mean, she was good in math before, but never *this* good." I didn't care. I was just glad she was good at roman numerals.

In the aftermath, each person in our family tried to wrap their heads around what had just happened. It felt like we'd been through combat and were trying to make sense of something impossible to make sense of. Like the experience of many combat veterans, it was difficult returning to the bewildering reality of people complaining about their cold espressos.

We emotionally held each other together, like lashing rafts in a storm. But we also went our own ways: Jeri gardened. Rachael hung out with her teenage friends. Julia withdrew into a world we didn't ask about. I read about miracles.

MIRACLES

As a scientist I find it hard to accept the concept of miracles. But what I saw in the ICU certainly looked like one. A couple of Julia's doctors also told me they thought that recovery from her state was a miracle—a *real* miracle. If a scientist observes an event but *rejects* the observation, is *that* scientific?

I read Graham Greene's *The Potting Shed,* the story of a man who experiences a miraculous event and struggles to fit it into his version of reality. I read C. S. Lewis's *Miracles: A Preliminary Study,* which faults science for a bias against the possibility of miracles. One book led to another, from Saint Augustine's *Confessions* to Erwin Schrödinger's *What Is Life?*.

Thirty books later, I was as confused as ever. Each one was interesting—fascinating, even—but none resolved my central question: Did I witness a miracle?

Although I didn't realize it until years afterward, the reason I found this question so important was that I needed to know whether Julia seemingly returned from the dead because she had a purpose for being here.

It may seem a bit odd to bring in Quentin Tarantino at this point, but please just go with it. In Tarantino's film *Pulp Fiction,* Jules, a gang henchman (played by Samuel L. Jackson), and his partner, Vincent (played by John Travolta), enter an apartment to collect a briefcase belonging to their boss, Marsellus Wallace (played by Ving Rhames). One of the guys in the apartment empties a loaded pistol at them, missing with every shot. Did Jules witness a miracle? Vincent and Jules disagree: Vincent believes it was due to sheer luck, while Jules believes it was divine intervention.

Early in the movie Jules "quotes" the Old Testament, Ezekiel 25:17:[2]

The path of the righteous man is beset on all sides by the iniquities of the selfish and the tyranny of evil men. Blessed is he, who in the name of charity and goodwill, shepherds the weak through the valley of darkness, for he is truly his brother's keeper and the finder of lost children.

And I will strike down upon thee with great vengeance

and furious anger those who attempt to poison and destroy my
brothers. And you will know my name is The Lord when I lay
my vengeance upon thee.

The marvel of Jules's not being shot prompts a transformation
in him, made apparent toward the end of the movie when he reflects
more deeply upon the fire-and-brimstone quote: "I never gave much
thought to what it meant—I just thought it was some cold-blooded
shit to say to a motherfucker before I popped a cap in his ass. But I saw
some shit this morning that made me think twice."

The philosopher Mark Conard[3] suggests that Jules's transformation is central to the movie's underlying theme: finding deeper purpose in a world in which values have fallen to the level of Big Macs
and Quarter Pounders, the Fonz, Arnold the Pig, Ed Sullivan, and
Marilyn Monroe. The "cold-blooded shit" that Jules cites speaks to the
self-transcending purpose of a person who, "in the name of charity
and goodwill, shepherds the weak." And to Jules, this purpose came
from God.

The first paragraph of Rick Warren's zillion-selling *Purpose
Driven Life* states, "If you want to know why you were placed on this
planet, you must begin with God. You were born by his purpose and
for his purpose."[4] Really? Is our purpose in life given to us by God or
can we create our own purpose? Let's return to the nineteenth century,
when centuries-old patterns of social, religious, and economic order
were bursting at the seams.

GOD

At one extreme is the German atheist Friedrich Nietzsche (1844–1900). At the other is the Danish Christian Søren Kierkegaard (1813–1855). Interestingly, both Nietzsche and Kierkegaard were considered the progenitors of the twentieth-century existentialist movement. Both also used basic stages of human development to describe their positions.

As described in chapter 3, Nietzsche's atheist hero starts out metaphorically as a camel (taking on the burdens and knowledge of the world), transforms into a lion (the experienced hero), slays the "thou shalt" dragon (rejecting society's and religion's values), and finally transforms into a child (the superman, the extreme hero transcending proscribed ethics and values).

Nietzsche famously attracted the likes of Adolf Hitler (who owned Nietzsche's walking stick) and Benito Mussolini. But a broad spectrum of authors (H. L. Mencken, George Bernard Shaw, Richard Wright), poets (Rainer Maria Rilke and Wallace Stevens), artists (Pablo Picasso and Salvador Dali), psychologists (Abraham Maslow, Carl Jung, Carl Rogers, and Rollo May), anarchists (Emma Goldman), U.S. presidents (Theodore Roosevelt and Richard Nixon), and of course, many philosophers (Martin Buber and Viktor Frankl, among many others) also read and admired his philosophy.

In general, people were attracted to Nietzsche's distaste for society's unquestioning adherence to state and religious control of beliefs and values (though ironically Hitler and Mussolini used this to their advantage), his praise of the artist and of creative endeavors, and his belief in the individual's freedom to choose one's values and destiny. He celebrated the person who abandoned social constraints and lived life to its fullest, saying, "The greatest enjoyment is—to live danger-ously! Build your cities on the slopes of Vesuvius!"[5]

Kierkegaard's hero, on the other hand, is a bit more like James Dean: the hedonic rebel who sucks the sensual marrow from the bone of life (what Kierkegaard calls the "aesthetic" stage). His model for this stage is Mozart's version of Don Juan, who becomes increasingly bored with his sexual conquests (apparently 1,003 in Spain alone).[6] As expected, Kierkegaard's aesthetic hero realizes he's living in an exis-tential vacuum—a rebel without a cause. Finding a cause in the secu-lar world, the rebel eventually lives a purposeful, ethical life.

This is where Nietzsche and Kierkegaard part ways. Whereas the Nietzschean hero rejects social norms to become a free thinker, Kierkegaard's hero rejects social norms after being pulled over the transom by God, becoming a "knight of faith." This leap into an unknown world is a leap of faith. Kierkegaard's example is the story of Abraham and Isaac, shared by Christians, Jews, and Muslims, where Abraham binds his beloved son and is ready to sacrifice him because God has ordered him to (at the last moment he's told that he's just being tested).

What Nietzsche and Kierkegaard present for us are the extremes of purposeful living: one extreme of rejecting societal values and find-ing one's own purpose (even though society might not understand it), the other extreme of rejecting societal values and living according to God's purpose (even though society might not understand it).

The *passion* of both extremes is impressive. The brilliance of H. L. Mencken, George Bernard Shaw, Richard Wright, Rainer Maria Rilke, and Pablo Picasso is fueled by their Nietzschean rejection of the status quo and by the personal creation of their identities.

To this day, however, whenever I grill steaks and feel the scorching heat of the coals, I recall the Kierkegaardian Saint Lawrence, a true "knight of faith" of the third century. Saint Lawrence made the prefect of Rome really angry by giving away much of the church's treasures to the poor. Ordered by the prefect to return the treasures, Saint Lawrence returned with the poor, the crippled, the blind, and the suffering and said that *these* were the real treasures of the church.

This made the prefect really, really angry, and he ordered Lawrence to be cooked on a barbecue. Really. While being grilled, Lawrence apparently joked, "I'm well done. Turn me over!" As I said, love the passion! Saint Lawrence is now the patron saint of both cooks and of comedians. No joke.

But Nietzsche's and Kierkegaard's ends of the spectrum seem a little . . . you know, extreme. We have, of course, Adolf Hitler traipsing through Bavarian forests with Nietzsche's walking stick. On the other hand, in a written testament, the 9/11 attacker Mohammed Atta made reference to the story of Abraham and Isaac.[7] Atta must have regarded himself as a "knight of faith."

So who is right? Do we need to choose? Must we reject God, as Nietzsche urges us, to find the true flame of our purpose? I don't believe so. Mother Teresa, Saint Francis of Assisi ("Every life needs a purpose to which it can give the energies of its mind and the enthusiasm of its heart"), and my well-done hero Saint Lawrence were each exemplars of self-transcending purpose.

The writer David Brooks points out[8] that religion gives us a "moral vocabulary," consistent with our cookbook metaphor. Talking about his own students at Yale University,[9] Brooks says that "they've been told all their lives 'come up with your own values' and my view is, if you're Nietzsche, maybe you can come up with your own values, but most of us, we can't . . . I do think it's important for them to at least think about closing in on a philosophy that has a name and a stream through history." Most philosophies that have names—the philosophical cookbooks of values—include the central tenet "Treat others the way you would like to be treated." This isn't a bad pillar from which to build your life purpose.

Must we, as Rick Warren and Søren Kierkegaard insist, "begin with God" to find our true purpose in life? Again, I don't believe so. There have been many purposeful atheists among us: Sinclair Lewis ("It is, I think, an error to believe that there is any need of religion to make life seem worth living"), Albert Einstein, Carl Sagan, Thomas Edison, Ayn Rand, George Bernard Shaw, Arthur C. Clarke, H. G. Wells, Ludwig van Beethoven, Wolfgang Amadeus Mozart, Mark Twain, Frank Lloyd Wright, and Paul Newman, to name a few.[10]

Must there be a greater meaning to our existence in order to have a self-transcending purpose? The existentialist philosopher Albert Camus, an atheist strongly influenced by Nietzsche, didn't think so. Taking exception to the old saying that "there are no atheists in foxholes," Camus was an active member of the French Resistance during World War II (fellow resisters around him were being captured, tortured into giving names of collaborators, and shot). And he had a strong purpose: the protection of France. "This country is worthy of the difficulty and demanding love that is mine."[11]

Camus didn't believe there was a universal meaning to life, which exposed a central existential question he states at the beginning of his book, *The Myth of Sisyphus:* "There is but one truly serious philosophical problem, and that is suicide."[12] If there is no meaning to life, he's asking, shouldn't we just kill ourselves? Camus concludes that, even in a futile, meaningless universe, life is indeed worth pursuing, but only if one lives it with purpose: "The struggle itself toward the heights is enough to fill a man's heart."[13]

THE AFTERLIFE

After giving a talk recently, I was approached by a minister from the audience who shook my hand and said, very kindly, "I'm sure that when you die, you'll go to the greatest country club with the best golf course ever made. You'll get to play every day!" I thanked him for his kind wishes but was a bit shocked. Could a religious person, who presumably spends a lot of time thinking about religious things, really believe that we spend eternity on a *golf course*? And if so, will I still slice?

In a book cheerfully entitled *Death,*[14] the philosopher Todd May points out that the way we think about death defines our approach to how we live. Most often, we avoid thinking about it; but when we do think about it, many of us believe in a religious idea of heaven (which, of course, can be seen as a way not only of not thinking about death, but of denying its existence altogether). In popular conceptions of heaven, we retain our consciousness of having been alive, get to catch up with dead friends and family, and possibly get a bird's-eye view of what's happening on the earth, all while spending eternity in the love and grace of our maker.

Is this really dying? It sounds more like a long vacation. If death is basically your life only better, why should we feel any urgency to get things done during *this* life?

The Hindu philosophy presupposes the reincarnation of the soul. A few years ago I spoke with a Vedanta Hindu guru in the foothills of the Himalayan Mountains and asked him how the concept of reincarnation affects Hindu culture. He laughed and said, "Well, look at India. We never get anything done!" When I pressed him for clarification, he answered, "If you know you're going to come back after you die, you don't feel like you need to finish things in this life."

The guru's words reminded me of *The Immortal*,[15] a short story by Jorge Luis Borges. It's about a Roman soldier entering a town through which flowed a river of immortality. He finds gnarled, repulsive, uncaring people in the decaying, dilapidated town. A person suffering after falling off a bridge was never rescued—someone would eventually "get around to it." The soldier realizes that the people were indeed immortal. With an infinite amount of time ahead of them, their empathy and compassion and urgency for learning and achievement were gone.

Chapter 3 introduced the headstone test, designed not to scare us but to stimulate urgency and a purpose. The Roman emperor and

Stoic philosopher Marcus Aurelius said to "not act as if you were going to live ten thousand years. Death hangs over you. While you live, while it is in your power, be good."

This has been long understood by economists. If you have $10,000, each dollar is worth proportionally less than it would if you only had five bucks. Yet we spend our *hours* as if they were an unlimited resource. As the Stoic philosopher Seneca said over two thousand years ago, "You are living as if destined to live for ever . . . You act like mortals in all that you fear, and like immortals in all that you desire!"

The headstone test is one way to stimulate urgency. Let's take it a step further.

What if we were to play a game called "No Afterlife"? Assume that when you die, your consciousness goes away *completely*. The atoms comprising your dead body eventually turn into other things. No heaven. No reincarnation. No golf course. No virgins. No nothing. Gone.

Now ask yourself, would you live your life differently? Elisabeth Kübler-Ross, the Swiss psychiatrist and author of *On Death and Dying,* concluded that "if all of us would make an all-out effort to contemplate our own death, to deal with our anxieties surrounding the concept of our death, and to help others familiarize themselves with these thoughts, perhaps there could be less destructiveness around us."[16]

COMPREHENDING OUR PERSONAL LEGEND

A few years after Julia had her second transplant, I was in Colorado, taking a long, solitary hike in the Rockies. After hiking all morning up a thirteen-thousand-foot mountain, I was looking forward to a quiet lunch at the top. Unexpectedly, I found one person already sitting there.

Grumbling silently that I wouldn't have the entire mountain range to myself, we exchanged a perfunctory "hi" and "nice view," then sat about twenty feet apart. But it felt odd—two strangers on a mountaintop eating sandwiches with no one within a five-mile radius—so before long we started up a conversation. It turns out he was an ICU physician.

We started talking about his interesting occupation, and I brought up the subject of Julia's "miraculous" recovery from a series of six heart attacks and lack of brain response. He looked into the distance and responded, "I saw a very similar case last year. An older man in our ICU had a sudden heart attack, and we couldn't revive him. After essentially calling it quits, he popped up and started talking to us. It really freaked us all out! Then he died a few hours later." He mused, "I think the body may have the ability to reboot itself in the way a seemingly dead computer can reboot. I can't understand how, but I've seen it."

I'm not an atheist. I claim neither faith nor disbelief in a god, which I guess makes me an agnostic. As a scientist I can live in a world that I can't comprehend. I'm used to this lack of comprehension and have spent much of my life reducing it. I know many scientists who are very religious—Christians, Jews, Muslim, Hindus, and others—and many who are not.

In my experience, not all scientists who believe in a god are stupid, and not all atheists are "brights" (as Richard Dawkins likes to call them, perhaps a tad smugly). Dawkins, to me, is like an ant telling his fellow ants that they can use the methods of observation and testing to better understand the true nature of the universe. To a very limited extent, yes. But remember, they're ants. Similarly, religious zealots are like ants telling everyone about the great ant in the sky who has a special plan for them. They don't know this. They're ants.

Like many scientists, I believe that scientific methods can make our ant-like lives better, but I also believe that these methods have their own limitations due to our ant-like inability to comprehend the larger reality of the universe. We fail, for example, to comprehend even the miracle of our own existence.

Any statistician could calculate that the odds of my daughter's survival—from the chances of receiving a new heart to surviving the transplant, to surviving many immune suppression–related illnesses, to surviving six consecutive heart attacks, to receiving a second heart transplant—were *infinitesimal*. The chances that you and I are here at all are even far more infinitesimal. We're pretty lucky ants.

This naturally makes me wonder whether our purposes are always lying within us, like the Greek daimon, awaiting discovery. In my own experience, I felt that finding my purpose was like a boat finding the right current and wind that then moves me effortlessly at a high speed. My only "job"—purposeful living—is to find this current and wind and to be able to steer within them.

In his beautiful book *The Alchemist,* Paulo Coelho writes about the importance of comprehending our "personal legend," which he

defines as "the path we decide to take that fills our heart with enthusiasm. It is the path of our dreams."[17]

Julia may have had, *and still has,* a personal legend. Her legend
now lives through me, and while this seems terribly unfair—that she
shouldn't be able to live out her *own* legend—I could make it even
less fair by ignoring her personal legend. So as I sail toward my own
harbor, I have my daughter with me in the boat. Like the person whis-
pering *memento mori* ("remember that you will die") into the ear of
the Roman general, Julia reminds me every day that life is short. So to
make the most of this journey—to be aligned with my purpose each
day—I need wind for my sails and a strong rudder.

Two

WIND AND A RUDDER

6

ENERGY

One swallow does not a summer make, nor one fine
day; similarly one day or brief time of happiness
does not make a person entirely happy.

ARISTOTLE[1]

BEING ALIGNED WITH YOUR PURPOSE IS A *DYNAMIC* ACTIVITY, NOT A one-shot accomplishment. It's a daily effort requiring energy and vitality. One of the world's experts on the subject of energy is Jim Loehr, a performance psychologist who works regularly with some of the top athletes (Jim Courier, Monica Seles, and many others) and business leaders in the world. At his Human Performance Institute (HPI)[2] in Orlando, Florida, Jim has seen millionaire executives breaking down and crying in his seminars because they're so unhappy. "My wife treats me like a stranger! My kids won't talk to me! Work isn't motivating anymore. I'm exhausted all the time!" Aw, poor millionaire executives! But Jim makes a good point: You'd think that millionaire executives would *automatically* be happy. Yet, despite their wealth, power, and status, they're often miserable because they lack motivation and energy.

Walking into Jim's home office during a recent visit to HPI, I saw a dozen or so books he was reading and stacks of written notes he was taking (in ink, by the way—he's a firm believer in the power of writing by hand). I spotted a copy of Mao Tse-tung's *Little Red Book* open on his desk. "I thought you were a staunch capitalist," I teased him. Jim just grinned. "I've been learning about brainwashing lately. I thought I'd better go to the source."

Jim is not your average seventysomething. With his wry smile and easy, ambling gait, he reminds me of James Coburn in *Our Man Flint*. I'm certain Jim could kill me with his bare hands. (So far he hasn't. But he could.) He works long hours at HPI, trains elite athletes and special forces teams, consults and speaks to executives of major corporations, and has written ten books. He conditions his body every day, which he demonstrated later in the afternoon by beating me in tennis 6–0, 6–0.

I asked him how he finds the time for all this. "It's not about time!" he said. "Time management is crap. Think about it. You get home after a grueling day at work. You reach for a drink and the newspaper. There's plenty of time to be engaged, but your spouse says, 'You're not here!' You respond angrily, 'Of course I'm here! I'm not traveling today—I'm here with you!' But you're not *here*. You're not present. You're not engaged. It's not about time. It's about energy management."

THE RIGHT ENERGY

When we think about our own energy, the concept seems pretty understandable and easy to rate. On a scale of one to seven, where has your energy level been over the past twenty-four hours? Have you been "on fire" or were you "drained"? Were you excited and engaged in what you were doing? Did your energy last the whole day, or did you run out of steam along the way? You may also want to ask yourself, Was it the right energy?

Roughly two thousand years ago, the Stoic philosopher Seneca wrote, "When a man does not know what harbor he is making for, no wind is the right wind."[3] Jim emphasizes that full engagement and performance occurs when one's energy is directed toward a specific purpose as opposed to being diffused through a fog of multitasking.[4] In other words, is your boat directed toward a specific harbor or is it simultaneously being pulled in lots of directions?

He also maintains that the "right energy" comes from positive emotions and values. For example, studies have shown that watching the performance of an elite athlete or artist can inspire positive emotions, which in turn create energy. Even during the normal course of a day, a benevolent act or a powerful presentation can create energy.[5]

Beauty can also be energizing. A study in Japan[6] found that walking in the woods (which the Japanese call "forest bathing") creates more energy than walking for the same period of time in an urban environment. The researchers of this study waved the "more research needed" flag, urging further research to study influences of "the stage of vegetation in the forest, as well as forest management and care." Sorry, researchers—you had me at *forest bathing*.

Another source of energy is the simple act of exercising your own human agency. Autonomy in our lives and in our work is a powerful generator of energy.[7] Think about it: working on an assignment that somebody else dumped on you wears you out, whereas working on one that you chose yourself results in greater engagement and better performance.

JIMMY CARTER AND AIMEE MULLINS: TWO REMARKABLE, PURPOSEFUL LIVES

I recently had the honor of speaking in Atlanta at Jimmy and Rosalynn Carter's Carter Center, an organization whose bold purpose is to "wage peace, fight disease, build hope." While touring the center's museum, I was struck by what a tough job the presidency is—neither your life nor your decisions are your own.

Many pundits and historians have written that Carter's difficult one-term presidency weighed heavily on him, and by some accounts he didn't take well to the loss of autonomy he experienced as president. After leaving the White House, however, it was clear that he was extremely well suited to being an ex-president. Unlike many of his peers before and since—who rode into a sunset of golf and stratospheric speaking fees—Jimmy (and Rosalynn) seemed to find a second wind, founding the Carter Center and taking on some of the most difficult political, health, and human rights challenges in the world.

Jimmy Carter grew up on a small farm in Plains, Georgia. Dreaming of a bigger and more exotic life, Carter applied and was admitted to the Naval Academy in Annapolis, where he met his future wife. After graduating in the top 10 percent of his class, he volunteered for the most hazardous of Navy services: submarines. While he was in Bermuda, British officials invited the sub's crew members to a party . . . but only the white ones. Carter successfully urged everyone on the submarine to refuse the invitation.

Carter's brilliant naval career was derailed when his father suddenly died, leaving a failing farm to his mother. Against Rosalynn's wishes, Carter left the bright and secure future of the navy to take care of the farm and his mother. He soon entered local politics, and well, the rest is history.

As I write this chapter, the ninety-one-year-old Carter has just announced that he has cancer that has spread to his brain. Meeting with the press to discuss his illness, he threw reporters a curveball, stating, "I would like the last Guinea worm [a particularly nasty parasite] to die before I do." He may well be dying, but he used his national exposure to push for a final end of Guinea worm disease, the incidence of which Carter Center efforts reduced from 3.5 million cases in 1986 to 126 in 2014!

After his cancer treatment, he said he intends to travel to Nepal to build more houses for Habitat for Humanity. Apparently no one told Jimmy Carter about the conservation of energy. He must have felt tremendous vitality and drive when he left the presidency and was suddenly free to work on *whatever* he decided to work on, with *whomever* he chose.

Psychologists use terms such as self-determination, autonomy, and intrinsic motivation to refer to decisions one makes for oneself, based on one's own values and purpose.

Aimee Mullins is one of the most self-determined people I've ever met. Born without fibulae in both legs, Aimee was told she would never walk and would likely spend the rest of her life using a wheelchair. To give Aimee an outside chance at independent mobility, doctors amputated both her legs below the knee—*on her first birthday*. Through her childhood, Aimee used heavy, painful prosthetic legs made of wood with metal hinges.

Aimee had a powerful "crossroads" experience while growing up.[8] "When I was fourteen, it was Easter Sunday, and I was going to be wearing a dress that I'd bought with my own money—the first thing I ever bought that wasn't on sale. A momentous event—you never forget it. I had a paper route since I was twelve, and I went to the Limited and bought this dress that I thought was the *height of sophistication*. Sleeveless safari dress, belted, hits the knee.

"As I'm coming downstairs, my father's in the living room waiting to take us to church. He takes one look and says, 'That doesn't look right. Go upstairs and change.' I was like, 'My super-classy dress? What are you talking about? It's the best thing I own!' He said, 'You can see the knee joint when you walk. It doesn't look right. It's inappropriate. Go change.' And something snapped in me. I refused to change. And it was the first time I defied my father. *I refused to hide something about myself that was true.*"

Later, while attending Georgetown University's prestigious School of Foreign Service, Aimee competed in NCAA track and field events against able-bodied athletes and was named by *Sports Illustrated* "one of the coolest girls in sports." Oh, I almost forgot. She's also one of the most beautiful women in the world, and a fashion model and actress.

Aimee has twelve pairs of prosthetic legs, including a pair of hand-carved wooden ones, and can now reign at *any* "height of sophistication," making cyborg-like transformations by choosing different legs. (I sometimes envy her when I'm jammed into a coach seat on an airplane.)

Aimee told me, "Changing my physicality is an overt, daily reminder of the power I have to shape myself in other ways. *I get to create and re-create the Aimee Mullins I want to be.*" Remember Nietzsche's metaphorical lion, who became a force of his own nature, slaying the dragon with "thou shalt" written on every scale? Aimee is a force of nature as well and has more energy than a pride of lions.

Jimmy Carter and Aimee Mullins demonstrate the ferocious energy that self-determined goals generate. And before you ask, "But how are they like me? One is an ex-president and the other is a globe-trotting model," remember that neither one started out that way. Jimmy Carter was born on a small farm in Georgia; Aimee was a first-generation immigrant from Allentown, Pennsylvania. There are lots of bright, attractive kids in the United States, but not many with the eudaimonic fire of Jimmy Carter or Aimee Mullins.

OTHER SOURCES OF ENERGY: THE BIG FIVE

I certainly don't put myself in the same category with Jimmy or Aimee, but I like to think of my own purpose as inspiring: helping others to create greater purpose in their lives, teaching my students as if each one were my own daughter, and being an engaged husband and father.

Every element of this purpose can easily burn me out. For example, teaching 250 University of Michigan undergrads each year requires hundreds of hours of preparation, frequently dozens of meetings a week, and then hours more writing recommendations to medical or graduate school, to internships, or to postgraduate jobs.

My first thought in considering how to stay aligned with this purpose was, "How will I find the time?" But as Jim Loehr says, it isn't about *time* management; it's about *energy* management. So I spent over a year studying ways I could increase my daily energy.

I began with physical activity and eating well, two areas that Jim Loehr's HPI program emphasizes—and then I added some more, all of which are supported by reputable research.

Activity. "Now wait," you might be asking. "How can *expending* energy give you more energy? After working hard all day, I'm exhausted!" In your physics class, you likely learned about a law called "the conservation of energy": that it can't be created or destroyed. We often carry the physicist's concept of energy to our subjective concept of our human energy. A wealth of scientific research shows that a broad range of exercise—from walking to resistance training to Pilates to water aerobics to boxing—increases our energy reserves.[9] Many studies have demonstrated the particularly important role physical activity can play in improving vitality among the elderly and those with various chronic diseases.

Eating. You've probably noticed how what you eat has a large and almost immediate effect on your energy. Eat a lot of fruits and vegetables? A vegan diet gives you more energy.[10] It also helps you lose weight, which—that's right—also results in more energy. Not ready for such an extreme diet? A "Mediterranean" diet (less red meat, more fish, fruits, and vegetables) has been shown to boost energy.[11] Jim Loehr's HPI intervention emphasizes a glycemic load diet, which focuses on the maintenance of a steady amount of glucose in your body. (We'll talk more about the Mediterranean diet and glycemic load in the next chapter.)

Sleep. Barely recognized a decade ago as a major factor in health, sleep is now getting a lot of attention from health researchers. A good night's rest is clearly associated with energy[12] but also with greater engagement and less absenteeism among employees, and with lower health-care costs. Unfortunately, at least a third of the adult population experiences insomnia.[13]

Presence. Another hot spot in research is mindfulness, which can include meditation, yoga, prayer, tai chi, and other contemplative practices that increase presence, or "being here now." In fact, the philosopher Eckhart Tolle dislikes the term *mindfulness* because, as he states, when present with the moment, the mind should be *empty,* not full. He prefers the term *presence.* Mindfulness training using meditation or yoga has been shown in numerous studies to increase energy and reduce stress.[14]

Creativity. Engagement in creative endeavors has been shown to enhance energy. An experiment conducted by a team of Swedish researchers found that individuals who were given tickets to films, concerts, art exhibits, or who sang in a choir demonstrated more energy than a control group did.[15] People who consider themselves creative also tend to have more energy.[16]

Based on available research evidence, five positive lifestyle practices shown to increase energy include *sleep, presence, activity, creativity,* and *eating.* In my life, the acronym SPACE provides a handy mnemonic, and each activity gives me the wind for my sails. But I needed something else, too. I needed a rudder to steer with.

7

WILLPOWER

Now don't say you can't swear off drinking;
it's easy. I've done it a thousand times.

W. C. FIELDS[1]

You might have seen the "marshmallow test"—a test of delayed gratification and willpower. An adult brings a young child into a room and gives them a marshmallow, telling the child that they could eat the marshmallow right away, but if they wait, they'll get *two* marshmallows. As you might imagine, the temptation drives the kids nearly insane and some simply cannot hold out. They smell the marshmallow. They try to divert their attention, but you can tell that they can't get the marshmallow out of their heads! The children look like they're in physical pain.

The ability of preschoolers to control themselves, it turns out, predicts their likelihood of being overweight or obese *thirty years later*.[2] Low willpower in childhood predicts adolescent smoking, school drop out, and teen parenthood. It also predicts a prediabetic condition known as "metabolic disorder" in adults, as well as substance abuse, sexually transmitted diseases, and even economic problems.

These demonstrations of the extraordinary stability of willpower over time are depressing to many behavioral scientists who try to help people make changes in their lives. Since eudaimonic well-being requires the willpower to align, and regularly *re*-align, with one's purpose, these findings are also relevant to us. How can we expect dynamic alignment with purpose when our will has been conditioned since childhood?

First, let's break some popular misconceptions about willpower.

SMOKING AND THE BEAR

Changing your behavior is hard. Changing your smoking behavior is *really* hard. Sigmund Freud had thirty operations for mouth cancer due to his cigar addiction. After his doctor strictly forbade further smoking, he wrote back, "I have not smoked for seven weeks since the day of your injunction. At first I felt, as expected, outrageously bad. Cardiac symptoms accompanied by mild depression, as well as the horrible misery of abstinence. These wore off but left me completely incapable of working, a beaten man. After seven weeks I began smoking again."[3]

One of the big issues in quitting smoking is temptation resulting from thoughts of cigarettes. The more that would-be quitters think about *not* thinking about them, the more they do. In psychology, this is called the "white bear" effect, from a phrase in Fyodor Dostoevsky's *Winter Notes on Summer Impressions:* "Try to pose for yourself this task: not to think of a polar bear, and you will see that the cursed thing will come to mind every minute."[4]

In the 1984 movie *Ghostbusters,* our heroes were asked to refrain from thinking about the form in which the malevolent spirit Gozer would come. One of the Ghostbusters, Ray, couldn't help himself, and Gozer came to destroy the earth as the giant Stay Puft Marshmallow Man (perhaps in tribute to the marshmallow test). The ability to suppress thoughts of an object—a marshmallow, a cigarette, or a polar bear—requires willpower.

For my doctoral dissertation in the early 1980s, I worked in a Veterans Administration (VA) hospital helping veterans quit smoking. At that time most of them smoked, and most said they wanted to quit but couldn't. I heard a lot of variations on "Well, it just takes *willpower* to quit—and I don't have any."

Many of the veterans had difficult lives, including addiction to other substances, and I wasn't at all sure I could do much to help. Working against me was the then-common notion that willpower was something you either were or weren't born with . . . and my vets weren't. They were telling me that as kids, they would have *failed* the marshmallow test.

John Wayne had willpower. Humphrey Bogart had willpower. These two icons of strength and courage were heroes to the World War II and Korean War vets at the hospital. And both Wayne and Bogart died from cigarette smoking. Even when Bogie was down to eighty pounds and breathing from an oxygen tank, he continued to puff away. Pure oxygen is a fire hazard (because it combines so quickly with many fuels), and smoking around an oxygen tank can lead to a huge explosion.

As I started working at the VA hospital, clinicians told me that patients were allowed to smoke in their rooms. The lung cancer and emphysema patients were often, like Bogie, breathing from oxygen tanks, so to avoid explosions, nurses would take long plastic tubing, stretch it outside of the room, insert a cigarette, and light it for them. As I said, quitting smoking is *really* hard.

So how to help? Until recently, the thinking among behavioral scientists was that even using the term *willpower* should be avoided at all costs. If willpower couldn't be changed, then every attempt should be made to "reattribute" the factors of success—from an unchangeable factor such as willpower to changeable factors such as learnable quitting skills.[5]

Willpower also had negative connotations for many social scientists because lacking it was seen to imply weakness. This victim-blaming implication, combined with the idea that willpower was more or less innate, kept the term in the closet for decades. Even one of the modern fathers of willpower research, Roy Baumeister, wrote that "the very notion that people can consciously control themselves has traditionally been viewed suspiciously by psychologists."[6]

Unfortunately for the social scientists, everyone else still used the term, so they had a hard time making it unpopular—possibly because it was real. Then some brave researchers, including Baumeister, started looking at willpower through a new lens. The big question facing them was whether willpower could be changed.

WILLPOWER AS A MUSCLE

Trials similar to the marshmallow test are also given to adults. Sitting up straight, speaking only in full sentences, refraining from swearing, or declining something tempting takes willpower. But psychologists have found that willpower acts in a similar manner to a muscle: it can be *depleted* after mental exertion, it can be *strengthened,* and it can be *fueled.*

Willpower can be depleted when one's ego is threatened—for example, by being berated or excluded. The ego threat requires mental exertion to reduce threat.

Are you a sports fan? How do you feel when your team wins? When they lose? Fans tend to connect their identities with their team. (Remember, the word is short for "fanatic.") It's not "They won," it's "We won." You're the "sixth person" on the basketball team. Your identity and your ego are involved in every game *your* team wins or loses.

French researchers Yann Cornil and Pierre Chandon[7] found, amazingly, that a community's average saturated fat consumption dropped by 9 percent on the Monday following a win on Sunday by their National Football League (NFL) team, and that a loss resulted in a 16 percent *increase.* And this result was measured across the entire community; the effect on hard-core fans would likely be even higher. (Imagine the class-action lawsuit against the NFL team: "You made us fat because you suck!")

Willpower-depleting mental exertion is also required when we're trying to remember something. In a Stanford University study,[8] students were given either a two- or seven-digit number. They were then instructed to walk down the hall to another room, where they'd be asked to recall the number. In the hallway they were offered a snack:

either fruit or chocolate cake. Fifty-nine percent of the students trying to remember a two-digit number chose the fruit, while only 27 percent of the students trying to remember the seven-digit number chose the fruit. Remembering the longer number required more mental exertion, and by the time the cake showed up, their willpower was depleted.

Consider the times when you have low willpower. Are you upset because your ego has been threatened through an argument with someone, a difficult discussion with your boss, or the loss of a team you identify with? Are you mentally exerting yourself? Have you been working too hard, overwhelmed by the challenges you face, having to keep too many things in your head? These events all cause a loss of willpower.

But what if you *always* have too many things in your head? What if you're just "hyper"?

HYPERACTIVITY AND WILLPOWER

We all know people who have a lot of energy but little or no willpower. Like a boat without a rudder, they can't maintain a course. Our society has a label for these people: annoying. The medical profession has other labels, such as attention-deficit/hyperactivity disorder (ADHD), obsessive compulsive disorder (OCD), or Tourette's syndrome (TS).

I was diagnosed as a child with TS. You might have heard of this condition—popularized by people who involuntarily shout obscenities in public places. This particular manifestation of TS is, thankfully, rare. My own version involved tics such as jerking my head, twitching muscles in my hands or face, or grunting, among other more creative elaborations. I also had a million thoughts racing through my head.

In the 1960s this condition wasn't well understood, and other than the occasional sadist (such as an unnamed second-grade teacher who'd make me wash my mouth out with soap or sit in a trash can for hours, in front of the whole class), adults would remark that I was "hyperactive" or, more generously, "had a lot of energy." In truth, I was annoying to others, and I could understand why. I was annoying to myself.

My body was a boat with sails unfurled on a windy day . . . but with no harbor and no rudder. Many adults simply thought I lacked the necessary willpower to stop the tics. "Just try not to twitch!" "Don't talk!" "Don't move!" Of course, trying not to do or even think about these things made it impossible *not* to.

The grown-up solution for my apparent lack of willpower, often the solution for children with ADHD and OCD, was medications. But they acted like an anchor to my sailboat. Even worse than sailing around with no rudder was being dead in the water.

In his book, *The Man Who Mistook His Wife for a Hat*, the late, great neurologist Oliver Sacks tells of a patient with Tourette's who was a weekend jazz drummer "of real virtuosity, famous for his sudden and wild extemporizations, which would arise from a tic or a compulsive hitting of a drum and would instantly be made the nucleus of a wild and wonderful improvisation."[9] Tourette's made him annoying; but it also made him a great jazz drummer. When Sacks gave him a drug to control the Tourette's, it quickly spelled the end to his tics . . . and to his brilliance. The drummer decided to stop taking the drug on weekends, and the jazz world was the better for it.

My parents saw a similar effect with me (my father had been a jazz musician himself) and, inspiring my eternal gratitude, let me twitch away. A more modern understanding of Tourette's syndrome finds that children with this condition are often massively creative. Howard Hughes, Dan Aykroyd, David Beckham, Samuel Johnson, and possibly Mozart all have or had it.

Creativity doesn't always equate with academic success, however. Finding myself close to flunking out of college, I envisioned a future as a very creative, very unemployed person. With tics and no willpower. In desperation I took up Transcendental Meditation my sophomore year. Initially, as with most people, I found that meditation was nearly impossible—so many random thoughts kept popping into my hyperactive head. But with time, TM eventually had a profound effect. Regular meditation gave me willpower, which, combined with exuberant energy, helped me perform well in school.

With both energy and willpower, I started to develop something I didn't previously have: a purpose. My purpose, in turn, gave me more energy and willpower. Amazing what can happen when you have wind in your sails, a rudder, and a harbor.

PURPOSE AS A SOURCE OF WILLPOWER

In a follow-up to the NFL study,[10] this time with French soccer fans, the researchers found that writing about core purposeful values completely eliminated the effect a loss had on willpower. Without values affirmation, watching a defeat increased fans' intentions to eat unhealthy foods. With values affirmation, however, watching a defeat *decreased* this intention: purposeful thinking increases willpower.

Based on the earlier discussion of eudaimonic versus hedonic values, you might wonder whether some values have a greater influence on willpower than others. Are some values more valuable than others?

In a beautifully designed and fun study by Aleah Burson and her colleagues,[11] ninety-two college students had their egos depleted by being told that they weren't picked by their classmates for a group project (a total lie, by the way; I feel so sorry for these students). Again, get your feelings hurt and you're likely to lose willpower and eat mass quantities. The researchers then divided the students into three groups. The control group was asked to write about their daily routine, the second group was asked to write about their *self-enhancing values* such as power, fame, wealth, or attractiveness, and the third group was asked to write about their *self-transcending values* such as empathy, support for others, or community.

Afterward, students in each group were given a bowl of cookies and asked to taste test the cookies as part of a consumer research study (another lie). The researcher said, "Eat as many as you want," and left the room. So, the researchers first threatened the students' egos, then wanted to test their willpower, measured by how many cookies they ate, but only *after* considering their self-transcending or self-enhancing values, or no values.

Students in the control condition ate an average of *eight* cookies! That, as I say to my students, is a lot of cookies. Chiding them, I ask, "Your feelings get hurt *and you eat eight cookies?*" They look back and say matter-of-factly, "Yes. What's your point?"

But here's the most important finding of the study: compared to the average of eight cookies eaten by the control group, those students considering their self-enhancing values ate an average of five, and those considering their self-transcending values ate an average of *three*. So, affirming *self-transcending*, purposeful values seems to produce the greatest surge in willpower.

What else can people do to enhance their willpower? Recent research suggests that the same influences of energy are also relevant.

OTHER SOURCES OF WILLPOWER

Sleep. A good night's sleep without medications boosts willpower. In a study of identical twins, the twin reporting fewer hours sleeping had, on average, lower willpower than the longer-sleeping twin. Inducing sleep deprivation in Chinese servicemen raised their levels of cortisol (the so-called stress hormone) and lowered their willpower.[12] Sleep-deprived adolescents are more likely to have lower willpower, which in turn, results in a higher rate of delinquency.[13] And among college students, both too little and too much sleep are associated with lower grades.[14]

Presence. Meditation boosted my willpower, and many studies show that other mindfulness-increasing practices such as yoga and tai chi do as well.[15] In addition, meditation has been shown to reduce aggressiveness among U.S. military veterans, to improve control of pain,[16] and to increase brain density in a region of the brain associated with emotional control.[17] Tai chi training has resulted in the reduction of ADHD symptoms.[18]

Activity. Physical activity plays a big part, too. For example, dieters decrease the amount of food they consume after exercising, particularly when the exercise is framed as "fun" versus "work."[19] As Stanford University lecturer Kelly McGonigal, author of *The Willpower Instinct,* writes, "According to the strength model of willpower, exercise should also temporarily exhaust willpower reserves. Over the long-term, however, it should lead to increased strength or endurance of the willpower 'muscle.'"[20]

Creativity. According to the psychologist Mark Runco, "The flexibility of creative persons is what gives them the capacity to cope with the advances, opportunities, technologies, and changes that are a part of our current day-to-day lives."[21] Improvements in creativity are associated with an important aspect of willpower—the ability to generate many possible solutions to a given problem.[22] After creativity training, researchers have demonstrated improvements in searching, retrieving, and integrating concepts from memory.[23] In fact, recent animal studies suggest that an enriched, stimulating environment not only leads to greater memory formation, but that this effect is transmitted to the next generation![24*]

Eating. Diet has a large influence on willpower. A study conducted by Matthew Gailliot and Roy Baumeister[25] found that restoring low glucose levels to normal increased control of attention, emotions, quitting smoking, managing stress, resisting impulsive behavior, and refraining from criminal or aggressive behavior. What and when you eat is therefore an important contribution to your willpower.

So the five key lifestyle factors leading to greater energy—sleep, presence, activity, creativity, and eating—*also* have a positive influence on willpower.

---

* The reason for excitement from these studies is that the transmission of memory formation is not through standard genetic transmission but through epigenetic changes to the genome.

To summarize, the dynamic process of aligning yourself with your life purpose requires energy and willpower: wind in your sails to move you forward, and a strong rudder to prevent being blown off course. And purpose, in turn, gives you more energy and willpower. What gives you more energy and willpower each day? Five positive lifestyle practices that can be summarized as SPACE—sleep, presence, activity, creativity, and eating. In my field, we like to put these relationships into box-and-arrow diagrams. Here's what I'm talking about:

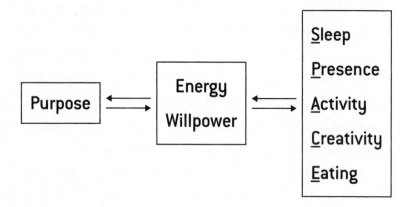

You can see from the diagram the reciprocal nature of purpose, energy, and willpower. It also illustrates a reciprocal relationship between energy and willpower and SPACE. We'll learn more about these and other influences of SPACE in the next section.

Three

SPACE

8

SLEEP

So I was walking down the street with my friend Pat
when this guy on an ostrich starts chasing us and we
race down this old stairwell and leap across train tracks
and I'm freaking out, like, "Holy shit, the subway is going
to hit us!" and the conductor has this crazy Skeletor grin
and I'm like, "Watch out, dude!" but Pat has turned into
my cousin Brad who isn't afraid of trains so we go into a
club and order a beer. Mmm, that beer sure tastes great.
And then Brad tries to sell me an illegal handgun and
I say no way and the bartender turns out to be Five-O
and so him and Brad chase me into the bathroom which
has a tunnel connecting to a huge circus tent full of
specially trained Jurassic stegosauruses moving in time
to house music blaring from two giant pole-mounted
conch shells and I sit in the front row next to my grade-
three teacher Miss Joanna and I'm like, "I always loved

you, Miss Joanna," and so she hands me a glass of water. Mmm, that water sure tastes great. And then Miss Joanna and I start to make out right there in the stadium and I'm like trying to get her top off and she's like, "No way, people are watching," and I'm like, "No they're not, come on, Miss Joanna," but then I realize that everyone really is watching and I have no pants on and Miss Joanna is gone and my girlfriend Kelly is in the audience and she's like, "I saw you with Miss Joanna," and I'm like, "That wasn't me, that was Pat," and she's like, "You're dumped, loser," and I'm like man I'm so stupid and then I see all the old letters I sent to Kelly strewn out in the dirt and I mope around for a while all agonized and then wonder, where's Miss Joanna?

JEFF WARREN, FROM A DREAM HE WROTE DOWN IN *THE HEAD TRIP*[1]

IT's BEEN FASCINATING TO WITNESS DURING MY LIFETIME THE exploration of other planets and objects in our universe. Still, it's odd that we have so little understanding of the planet resting right on top of our shoulders. Want to explore a truly amazing object? Try the brain. And one of the brain's best-kept secrets is how we spend a third of our lives: asleep.

When I was a college student in the 1970s, we didn't talk about sleep. We didn't spend much time doing it, either. In fact, until the end of the previous century, little attention was paid to the health benefits of sleep, or the problems caused by too little (or, occasionally, too much) of it. We still don't respect even the most basic knowledge of sleep patterns. For instance, for the convenience of teachers and parents, we make children start learning too early in the day, before their brains begin to function properly.

When analyzing data for HealthMedia, a wellness company I founded in 1998, we consistently saw large impacts of poor sleep on health problems, health-care costs, and absenteeism. Across the United States, the pattern of insufficient sleep matches almost identically with the prevalence of obesity and diabetes. Poor sleep is a risk factor on the order of cigarette smoking, poor diet, or sedentary behavior. As I mentioned in the previous chapter, a good night's sleep also amps up energy and willpower.

We require sleep to restore our immune system and to enhance brain plasticity—changes in neural pathways that develop due to our behavior, the environment, our emotions, and our thoughts. The vast majority of animals require sleep, but the amount varies widely. Horses and elephants sleep about three hours a day, lions more than thirteen. Bats sleep about twenty. Dolphins, who need to be conscious to breathe, put only half of their brains to sleep at a time—they're always "half-awake"!

Deprived of sleep, we die. Without it, a rat will die in ten to twenty days. We don't know how long it would take to kill a human with sleep deprivation, but it has undoubtedly occurred through torture. The holder of the longest scientifically recorded period of voluntary sleeplessness without stimulants is Randy Gardner, a sixteen-year-old high school student in San Diego, California. He stayed awake for 264 hours. Before he finally dozed off, Gardner had problems with mood, concentration, short-term memory, paranoia, and hallucinations.

HOW MUCH SLEEP?

Humans normally need seven to eight hours in a twenty-four-hour period. When we stray far outside that range, trouble begins. As mentioned previously, college students whose average sleep falls above or below that range have lower grade point averages. While many individuals (particularly my college students) *think* they can get by on less sleep, the vast majority of us require *at least* seven hours to optimize energy and willpower.

Thomas Edison, among others, did not agree. He argued that eight hours of sleep is a "deplorable regression to the primitive state of the caveman."[2] In 1662 Robert Boyle, the scientist and father of modern chemistry, created a "wish list" of things he hoped science would one day achieve. In addition to "The Prolongation of Life," "The Recovery of Youth, or at least some of the Marks of it, as new Teeth, new Hair colour'd as in youth," and "The Art of Flying," he longed for "Freedom from Necessity of much Sleeping."

Frequent napping can indeed reduce the need for one long period of sleep. Recent research has demonstrated that naps of no longer than six minutes produce marked improvements in memory performance and can, in fact, replace much longer periods of genuine shut-eye.

Given the positive impact of naps, we now have at JOOL Health, a well-being company I founded in 2015, a nap and meditation room for employees. Visitors to our offices look twice when they notice the room's solid-glass wall. At first some employees feared that it would be embarrassing to sleep (let alone snore or drool) in front of others and requested blinds, but they quickly got used to it. Employees using the snooze room don't seem self-conscious about napping, and passing employees simply ignore them. Although the room is very popular—especially for afternoon siestas—so far no one has abused the privilege by sawing logs all day, throwing slumber parties, or wearing bunny slippers.

Some cultures have adopted more fluid periods for sleeping and waking. Many hunter-gatherer cultures, for example, sleep for brief periods many times a day. Their style of sleep also differs from most of ours: in large groups in exposed locations, with minimal bedding. At least one person always stays awake, for protection against animal or human predators. This "polyphasic" pattern is considered completely normal and appropriate among these cultures. It's also normal for other creatures. In fact, polyphasic sleep is, according to researchers Scott Campbell and Patricia Murphy, "the rule, rather than the exception, across the entire animal kingdom."[3]

Our modern "monophasic" pattern generally involves sleeping in beds, alone or in pairs, out of sight and earshot of others, at regular times of day. Western cultures with predominantly monophasic sleep patterns frown upon napping. But employers might frown a bit less if they found that their napping employees were more productive during the day. Since it's often difficult to get sufficient sleep during the night, nap rooms may prove to be an effective approach to optimizing energy and willpower. Thomas Edison was not exactly a sloth and dullard. Nor were Leonardo Da Vinci, Nikola Tesla, Buckminster Fuller, or Napoleon—all frequent nappers.

WHAT IS SLEEP, ANYWAY?

Sleep can be broken into a number of measurable phases, each with its own function. I won't go into great detail here, but the basics are relevant. First, the transitions into ("hypnogogic" state) and out of ("hypnopompic" state) sleep are important, since both appear to be important states where creative ideas are generated. Champion snoozer Thomas Edison would begin his nap in a chair with a metal plate placed on the floor underneath his hand, which held a ball bearing. When he'd doze off, his hand would relax and the ball would drop with a clang, waking him. He'd then write down whatever he'd been thinking about at the time. He claimed that this process was a significant source of his ideas and his over one thousand patents.

I've personally found the stretch between 5:00 A.M. and 6:00 A.M. (the hypnopompic state) a fertile and creative time. I keep a notepad or my smartphone on the nightstand for recording ideas, which I then review when I'm fully awake. Many aren't worth further consideration (the design of a hat with holes for my ears didn't seem worth pursuing), but many are (a book about purpose in life).

Once asleep, breathing becomes slower and more regular and body temperature drops. Your eyes roll gently back and forth while all attention to the external world falls away. Connections among different regions of the brain also diminish. This early but deep period is called slow-wave sleep.

The benefits of slow-wave sleep are rest and repair of the body. Growth hormone is released and cortisol, the so-called stress hormone, which suppresses the immune system, is reduced. Facts and knowledge gathered during the day are encoded into long-term memory.

The next phase, occurring intermittently and increasing in length, is REM (rapid eye movement) sleep. Ninety-five percent of dreams happen during this phase. (Dreams also occur during slow-wave sleep, but they're far less vivid and harder to remember.)

Brain activity during REM is similar to what we experience while awake. But rather than taking in and encoding facts, REM is the period when the brain makes creative associations and consolidates skills into memory. And the roughly two hours of dreaming that we do each night play a role in these functions.

WHY DO WE DREAM?

Dreams are among the coolest and most bizarre aspects of our lives. Take the one at the beginning of this chapter. While awake, Jeff Warren probably entertains no thoughts of making out with his third-grade teacher. So why did he dream it? Was it, as Freud might suggest, the fulfillment of a secret wish?

I doubt it.

Jeff's dream was more likely a "virtual rehearsal" for a similar, though perhaps less outrageous, event in real life. It could have been related to a person that he wanted to make out with, but he wasn't sure how it would go. Researchers believe that the extreme simulations we encounter in dreams build skills, create warning signals, and stimulate new creative connections.

Here are a few of my own recurring dreams and my interpretations:

- teaching my class stark naked (reflects a worry about preparation)

- running but not able to gain any speed (a concern over something I'm trying to accomplish)
- climbing an enormous ladder, only to have it fall backward (a practical, physical skill related to balance)
- making out with my second-grade teacher in a trash can (I'm kidding)

The interpretation of symbols in dreams was popularized by Sigmund Freud in his famous book *Interpretation of Dreams*.[4] According to Freud, flying represented repressed sexual desires and phallic shapes represented the penis. (Although the frequent smoker apparently did say that "a cigar is sometimes just a cigar.") The psychologist Hans Eysenck criticized Freud as "a genius, not of science, but of propaganda, not of rigorous proof, but of persuasion, not of the design of experiments, but of literary art."[5] Freud apparently didn't care to waste much time testing his theories.

Symbolism in dreams actually goes back thousands of years. An ancient papyrus document dating to 1220 BC, now in the British Museum, contained "The Dream Book," which among other interpretations claimed that when a man dreams that his bed is catching fire, he is "driving away his wife," whereas when he dreams of mating with a cow, he's obviously "spending a happy day in his house." I'll leave the psychosocial implications of those to others.

Regardless of their content, the connections made in dreams clearly generate new and complex ideas. Einstein claimed that the special theory of relativity came to him in a dream. The complexities of a sewing machine (a very intricate device) came to Elias Howe in a dream. Dmitri Mendeleev dreamt up the periodic table of elements. I find organic chemist Friedrich August Kekulé's dream especially delightful: "Atoms were gambling before my eyes . . . all twining and twisting in a snake-like motion. Look! What was that? One of the snakes had seized hold of its own tail, and the form wormed mockingly before my eyes."[6] Kekulé had just dreamt up the structure of the benzene ring.

As I said, dreams are cool. Like Thomas Edison, me, and many others, you might consider putting a notebook or other recording device at your bedside and recording your dreams and thoughts. You'll likely forget them if you don't.

SIMPLE TIPS FOR IMPROVING YOUR SLEEP

Here are some simple tips that you may want to try. (I'll present tips in each of the SPACE chapters—they're based on scientific knowledge and have been used successfully by real people.)

What keeps us up at night? Plenty of things: *behavioral factors,* such as weight, inactivity, caffeine, and alcohol; *environmental factors,* such as irregular work schedules, electronic media, light, and noise; and *emotional factors,* such as worry and stress. With this understanding, here are some tips developed by experts and former insomniacs that might help you sleep better.

YOUR BEHAVIORS:

- Your bedroom is a special room: it's the sleeping room. Oh, and if the kitchen table, living room rug, hearth in the den, and basement Ping-Pong table are all occupied, it can also be used for sex. As such, use it *only* for sleep and sex. Not for television, e-mailing, video games, or for the many other technologies that have invaded this sacred space.

- Computers and other screens emit a blue light that suppresses the production of the sleep hormone melatonin. Ideally you should turn them off at least an hour before bedtime.

- You may think that alcohol makes you sleep more easily. Unfortunately, going to sleep drunk produces what has been likened to a series of minihangover events through the night. Normal sleep cycles are interrupted, leaving you drained the next day.

- For that matter, try to limit how much you drink of *anything* before bedtime, to minimize late-night bathroom trips. Sometimes these can't be helped (hello, Mr. Prostate!), but of course it's good to limit the number of times you need to get up.

- Melatonin. This hormone can help you fall asleep quicker and wake up refreshed. It's cheap, and you can buy it over the counter at any pharmacy.

- Physical activity is good for sleep, but not if it's too close to bedtime. Your body gets revved up right after physical activity, and you want to be calm before going to bed.
- Don't go to bed hungry—the siren song of the refrigerator can be hard to tune out.

YOUR ENVIRONMENT:

- Unless you work the night shift, try to get plenty of natural light during the day. Then keep things dark at night. This supports the circadian rhythm: the internal clock that regulates your wake-sleep cycle.
- Keep your bedroom quiet, dark, comfortable, and cool.
- Try turning off the sound, and even the vibrator, on your phone. You may not be consciously aware that those little beeps and buzzes are actually disrupting your deeper sleep patterns, but they may be.
- Have pets? They may be your best friend, but that doesn't mean you should be sharing a bed with them. When they're restless (and they generally are), *you're* restless. They also generate heat—another factor that might be keeping you awake.
- Earplugs help. Not only do they limit external noise, they also magnify the sound of your breath, helping you focus on your rhythm of breathing instead of your hectic life.

- Sleep experts suggest keeping your room between sixty and sixty-seven degrees Fahrenheit. Try nudging the thermostat down a tad and see if it leads to better sleep.

- It may be time for a new pillow. Unlike the bad old days, when the only options seemed to be marshmallow and cinder block, pillows now come in a bewildering variety of shapes, sizes, and levels of firmness. Test-drive a few and don't give up until you find the perfect match for your head, neck, and back. Years ago I found the perfect pillow—so perfect that I named him (yes, he's a "he"). His name is Bill and he's my friend. Bill makes my wife jealous. Really.

YOUR EMOTIONS:

- Push distractions out of your mind by thinking about something upbeat about your previous or upcoming day. Start with your morning and slowly, meticulously work your way through all the minute details of the day. Sound boring? That's the point.

- Stop your mind's buzzing in bed by listening to white noise (sound energy evenly distributed across the audio spectrum). And yes, there's an app for that. Just search for "white noise" in your app store. It's like the sound of the ocean, the wind in the trees—a constant humming or droning sound that masks distractions and eases your mind.

- Try curling your toes: hold for a few seconds, then uncurl them. This exercise helps to relax your muscles and diverts your attention from whatever is keeping you up.

- Control your breath by inhaling softly through your nose through a count of four, holding it through a count of seven, and exhaling completely through a count of eight. And repeat. And repeat.

- Finally, my SPECIAL SECRET NINJA TIP: When Julia was alive, Jeri and I used to stay up a lot worrying about her. One simple strategy worked: the BBC. Tuning into the BBC and playing it just above the threshold of hearing for thirty to forty-five minutes (we have a radio with a sleep timer) would shift our minds from Julia to the international cricket scores, which would of course put us into an immediate coma: "India won by fifty-nine runs . . . England won by five runs . . . New Zealand won by eight wickets . . . Australia won by an inning and forty-six runs . . ." Zzzzzzz.

Sleep heals your body and gives you more energy, but it also rests your mind so you have more self-control upon waking. Another way to rest and refocus your mind is through becoming more present and mindful, which we'll discuss in the next chapter.

9

PRESENCE

If you just sit and observe, you will see how restless
your mind is. If you try to calm it, it only makes it worse,
but over time it does calm, and when it does, there's
room to hear more subtle things—that's when your
intuition starts to blossom and you start to see things
more clearly and be in the present more. Your mind
just slows down, and you see a tremendous expanse
in the moment. You see so much more than you could
see before. It's a discipline; you have to practice it.

STEVE JOBS[1]

MIDSUMMER. I'M RIDING UP A SKI LIFT TO THE TOP OF VAIL MOUN-
tain with Tenzin Priyadarshi, a Buddhist monk who's also president
of the Dalai Lama Center for Ethics and Transformative Values at the
Massachusetts Institute of Technology (MIT). I was asked to join Tenzin for a mountaintop discussion about purpose in life for a group of
people interested in well-being. With my jeans and Blue Öyster Cult
"Don't Fear the Reaper" T-shirt and his flowing red monk robe and
beads, we make an odd couple.

Knowing Tenzin can't really go anywhere without falling a hundred feet, I pepper him with questions. He answers them politely and
thoughtfully despite their crushing naïveté. Imagine a kind teenager
responding to questions from an admiring five-year-old:

"Do you meditate, Tenzin?" (As if I asked him, "Do you play
with toys?")
"Yes, twice a day."
"Oh, I meditate too!" ("I play with toys, too!")

"That's wonderful."

"I meditate for twenty minutes a day. How about you, Tenzin?" ("My mommy lets me play after I take a nap.")

"Well, this morning I started my meditation at four thirty A.M. It went for roughly two hours. I'll meditate again this afternoon for that long."

"Oh. Uh. Do you have a mantra? I have a mantra." ("I have a truck!")

By now I figure it's fifty-fifty that he'll jump off the lift and take his chances. Instead, he gives me a benign smile.

"Actually, this morning I was meditating on my own death."
"Oh."
"This afternoon, I'll focus on my decomposition," he says casually, as if he were going to play an Xbox game.
"Oh."

I can't explain why, but the look Tenzin gave me reminded me of the moment in *Blade Runner* when Batty, the godlike android (played by Rutger Hauer), tells Deckard (played by Harrison Ford), "I've seen things you people wouldn't believe. Attack ships on fire off the shoulder of Orion. I watched C-beams glitter in the dark near the Tannhauser gate. All those moments will be lost in time, like tears in rain."

Meditating on his death for months in a cave, Tenzin may well have seen "C-beams glitter in the dark near the Tannhauser gate." He isn't an android like Batty, but he is otherworldly and I'm certain that his brain doesn't work the way mine does. (Then again, I was the one with the "Don't Fear the Reaper" T-shirt.)

A year earlier I was in Delhi, India, for a public health meeting. The meeting went fine, but I grew antsy and wanted to learn more about the India I'd pictured in my mind. So I took a weeklong detour, north to Rishikesh, at the foothills of the Himalayas on the famed Ganges River. Rishikesh is considered a holy city to Hindus and nick-named "the yoga capital of the world." The Beatles wrote most of their *White Album* there in 1968 while visiting the ashram of Maharishi Mahesh Yogi, who developed and promoted Transcendental Medita-tion (TM for short). I was told that the ashram has since been aban-doned and filled with monkeys and possibly a panther.

Just north of Rishikesh, I met with a Vedanta Hindu guru (which simply means "teacher") and his protégés and discussed medi-tation and moksha (the Hindi word for freedom achieved through self-transcendence), among other subjects. "There are over two hundred forms of meditation, appropriate for different people in different situ-ations," the guru told me. He warned me that some practices might be dangerous for me because "you're simply not ready." He wouldn't tell me *which* ones. Okay, I get it. I'm not enlightened. They must have seen me at the bar the evening before.

One of the meditation practices—involving long chants with other practitioners—sounded very much like Gregorian chants I'd heard. My guru laughed when I told him that. "Ah, yes, it's *just the same*! There's a vibration created by the chant—feels good, doesn't it?"

"Yes!" I answered. "Like when I was taught 'om chanting,'

there's a vibration created above the roof of my mouth. It feels as if I'm giving my innermost brain a nice massage."

"Exactly!" he exclaimed.

Throughout the week, I practiced breathing meditation, mantra-based meditation, chanting, and yoga and explored the possibility that I might have spiritual channels spinning inside of me (called chakras). We wore white pajamas all day. My guru wore the standard guru uniform but didn't really look the part. He looked like an engineer, which he formerly was. No long, tangled hair and beard. No far-off look or goofy grin. He was intelligent and funny (we laughed a lot), and he was completely engaged in the moment.

In a word, he was *present*.

WHAT IS PRESENCE?

Jon Kabat-Zinn, a leading researcher of mindfulness practices, defines presence as "paying attention in a sustained and particular way: on purpose, in the present moment, and non-judgmentally."[2] This is exactly what I felt when talking with Tenzin Priyadarshi in Vail and with my guru in northern India. Presence. Attentiveness.

The word *mindfulness* is often used to describe this feeling, but as discussed previously, presence really occurs *when your mind is empty* and you're completely attentive to what's going on right now. The "right now" could be the conversation you're having with someone. It could be a mantra (a simple word, phrase, or sound) you're repeating. It could be your breathing. It could be your cadence as you walk.

Presence is achieved through meditation, yoga, qigong, tai chi, and many other practices. But it can also be found in gardening, lovemaking, and even sports. Prayer *can* create presence if one isn't focused on past or present events ("I'm sorry for this or that" and "I hope you'll help me with this or that" are not here-and-now prayers). There are, however, forms of prayer that are very similar to the practice of meditation. What's important is that the activity allows you to be in the present moment.

When the 1970s tennis star Björn Borg was asked what he was thinking about when playing his very best tennis, he answered, "Nothing." A person is present, in the moment, when her head isn't filled with thoughts of the past ("Why did or didn't I do that?") or the future ("What will I do? How will I get this done?"). Unfortunately, most of us have nearly constant thoughts of the past or the future. We're replaying an argument we had with someone, convincing ourselves of how right we were. Or we're thinking about what we'll eat for lunch, or what we'll say to our teenage son.

But do you ever find yourself in a place where time just . . . goes away? Where you're in a "flow state"? Is it when you're writing? Painting? In a fun conversation? Gardening? Walking in the woods? Are there times when the birds sound louder? The flowers smell better? The evening sky looks more spectacular? Athletes talk about being "in the zone": when the golf hole looks a foot wide, when the basketball hoop seems three feet wide. This is presence.

There are moments in our lives when time seems to slow down—not the way it slows during an excruciating lecture, sermon, or dental procedure, but when we become more keenly aware of sensory experiences, feelings, and bodily states. To a jazz musician, it's when the notes flow like magic; to a quarterback, it's when a play slows down and the movements of others are clearer and more predictable. Again, this is presence, and researchers have found that it can be increased through meditation.[3]

MEDITATION

Studies show that the regular practice of meditation delivers consistent, positive effects on our physical and mental well-being. A particular type of meditation, called "loving-kindness meditation," has been shown to enhance self-transcendence and purpose in life, and even to repair your DNA. (You'll find instructions for this meditation later in this chapter.)

Depending on the specific practice, and there are many of them, meditation can increase energy[4] and willpower,[5] reduce insomnia,[6] improve diet,[7] and enhance creativity.[8] A recent well-controlled study found that even simple "breathing meditation" decreased post-traumatic stress disorder (PTSD) in U.S. military veterans.[9] If in the research literature you replaced the name of a drug with the word *meditation*, the pill would be called "magic" and probably outsell Viagra, Zocor, and Flintstones Vitamins combined.

Meditation was very popular in the 1970s, when the Beatles and other notables were taking up the practice. Now, after stagnating for decades, it's seen a massive resurgence in both practice and in research.

Many forms of meditation have been tested, and as I said, there are lots of ways to meditate.

"Focused-attention meditation" is as simple as observing your breathing or repeating a simple sound or "mantra." A mantra is a sound or vibration that allows you to enter a state of meditation. You can focus on a word of your choice (like *love* or *one*) or search online for "meditation mantra examples." There are lots of words and sounds commonly used as mantras, most coming from ancient Sanskrit words, including the classics *om* and *om mani padme hum*. Other mantras include *ah* and *hum*. There are other mantras that are easy to find online, and you may want to listen to a few.*

Mantras, including the aforementioned ones, can be repeated regularly to yourself, without the need of embarrassing yourself in a crowd. I usually meditate in my home or office, but I've also meditated in cabs, hotel rooms, lobbies, airplanes, on seashores and mountaintops, and in many other places. Just pick a space where you won't be interrupted.

Here is a simple, step-by-step approach to meditation using either your breathing or a mantra:

---

* Amazingly, there are visual representations of these sounds. In India, my guru informed me that the clear and practiced mantra chants of Buddhist monks can create elaborate patterns in pools of sand. You can find videos of this phenomenon online. This isn't magic but, like the effect of an opera singer shattering a glass, illustrates the power of sound waves. And even without the sand, just sitting with others chanting a mantra out loud can produce a beautiful resonance that *feels* good. Anyone in a choir or barbershop quartet knows what I'm talking about.

The sounds themselves are meaningless to most of us, but they provide the vehicle for entering a meditative state. Some meditation trainers insist on the proper pronunciation of mantras, but many don't. Deepak Chopra, for example, points out that concern over pronunciation can actually undermine the meditation process.

- Find a comfortable place to sit, either in a chair or on the floor. Close your eyes. Take a few moments to just be, just *noticing* the sounds, smells, and feelings. Allowing yourself to settle down, turn your attention to your breathing.

- Notice the way your body automatically, effortlessly inhales and exhales.

- Don't try to manipulate your breath in any way. Notice the feeling of air moving in and out of the nose and the easy, natural way your body moves.

- If you're using a mantra, begin repeating it slowly in your head.

- Your mind will occasionally wander away from your breath or mantra (depending on whichever you're focusing on). This is actually an important part of meditation. As unwanted thoughts, feelings, or sensations intrude, simply acknowledge them and let them percolate up like bubbles rising in a pool of water. Then gently let your attention return to your breath or mantra.

- When you're finished meditating, spend a minute or so with your eyes shut before opening them, rising slowly, and going back to your daily routine.

- Consider starting with this exercise for about five minutes each day. If meditation helps clear and rest your mind, you can increase your sessions over a couple of weeks to twenty minutes twice a day.

The technique I just described may not work for you. Luckily there are many instructional sites on the Web. Focused-attention meditation (on your breath or a mantra) is only one form, but it's quite simple and easy to maintain.

If you're uncertain about which mantra to use or how to get into meditation, I'd recommend a teacher. If you have a Buddhist center in the neighborhood, that can be a good place to start. Transcendental Meditation (TM) offers extensive training and helped me get started. Their focus is to provide a simple road to meditation for the average person. It's not cheap, but I know from my own personal experience that the money was well spent. I remember paying $75 to learn TM in 1974, but that was when a bottle of Château Lafite Rothschild was $25 (also money well spent).

Meditation is often viewed as a method of relaxation and stress reduction, and many research studies demonstrate this effect. Beginning meditators find these relaxing effects quickly, and they can expect to feel calmer and to sleep better. But as the meditation progresses, the practitioner can expect greater alertness and less mind wandering during the day while requiring less sleep at night.[10]

As I mentioned earlier, I started meditating as a sophomore in college. I credit it with keeping me in school and helping me get good grades. It allowed me to quiet my very noisy mind and to become more alert, aware, and awake during the day.

MOVEMENT PRACTICES

As a visiting professor at Peking University in China, I spend a fair amount of time in large Asian cities. In Hong Kong, for example, I'll often wake up jet-lagged around 4:00 A.M. and stroll through the city. In their beautiful urban parks, well before daybreak, I'll notice groups of people—young to very old—moving and breathing rhythmically together.

The beauty and power of qigong and tai chi—the two most popular traditional Chinese mindful movement practices—are far better seen than described. Watching a group of twenty women in their eighties slowly turn toward you like the Shaolin monk Caine (played by noted non-Asian David Carradine) from the 1970s series *Kung Fu* is a little like watching a panther yawn: at once beautiful and frightening.

Qigong is thousands of years old and has always focused on "inside energy flow."[11] It can be practiced sitting, lying, standing, or moving and is considered easier to practice than tai chi, which was invented by a retired army general as a martial arts style in the seventeenth century. Tai chi now has many gentler styles, including the "Yang style" and "Sun style." Both of these movement-based therapies are now primarily used to stimulate energy and willpower and are used increasingly to lessen disease and chronic pain.

Probably the most popular movement therapy in the Western world is yoga, a set of diverse practices that include physical, breathing, relaxation, and meditation exercises. Like many others, I've popped into the occasional yoga class when on vacation or at a fitness center. I'm sorry to report that my experiences haven't been pleasant: being twisted into a pretzel, then told to balance on one foot and to hold this "pose" alongside many other far more flexible people for what felt like an hour. When my body was ready to burst into flames, the instructor gently said, "Make sure to breathe!" I'd leave with a week of knee problems and a bruised ego.

When mentioning my experiences to practitioners of yoga, I usually get, "Oh, but you just had a bad instructor. You should try *my* instructor!" For me, this is like eating lamb (which I've tried dozens of times and still can't stand). People always say, "But you should try *my* lamb!"

I am trying, however, to like yoga. At JOOL Health we have a yoga room and often bring in a really good instructor who has our employees stretching, balancing, twisting themselves into reef knots—and breathing. I *should* like yoga. Scientific research has shown truly remarkable outcomes from the practice, from reductions in stress and anxiety to improvements in sleep, energy, willpower, and general well-being.[12]

If you are, or know of, a cancer survivor, please note an excellent recent study[13] assigning two hundred breast cancer survivors to either twelve weeks of twice-weekly, ninety-minute hatha yoga sessions or to a control group who were put on a waiting list to receive the yoga classes. After three months the yoga group not only had more energy but also less chronic inflammation. The markers of inflammation the researchers measured[14] are related to frailty, disability and death.

THE POWER OF THE HIVE

Let's picture ourselves in one of these yoga classes. I can imagine two scenarios. One would be a group of cancer survivors who didn't really know each other but instead used their mats as if they were separate islands. The other group would get to know each other by name, support struggling members, and end their last class with a tearful group hug of hope, strength, and resilience.

The researchers of the yoga study were justifiably interested in *isolating* the possible effect of yoga (which they found), so they were probably relieved to report that "yoga participants did not report the changes in social support [not yoga] that would be expected if support were the key mechanism." In other words, the "active ingredient" that benefited the cancer survivors was not the social support but the yoga itself. But what would have happened in the second scenario, where there was a collective energy created by the group?

When individuals come together to create a community, their energy, willpower, and eudaimonic well-being are amplified. In their "hive hypothesis," psychologist and author Jonathan Haidt and his colleagues suggest that such groups create self-transcendence: "The most effective moral communities (from a well-being perspective) are those that offer occasional experiences in which self-consciousness is greatly reduced and one feels merged with or part of something greater than the self."[15]

The collective energy and purpose of the "mindful hive" allows the individual to lose one's ego, whether group chanting in northern India; doing Qigong in a Hong Kong city park; doing yoga in a Columbus, Ohio, cancer center; parading giant handmade puppets on Main Street in Ann Arbor, Michigan; singing in a Washington, DC, gospel choir; or dancing to the zydeco rhythms in a Lafayette, Louisiana, town square.

There are many ways to incorporate presence and mindfulness into your life short of becoming a Buddhist monk. Like sleep, the benefits of even short bursts of the practices presented in this chapter can significantly improve your energy and willpower.

LOVING-KINDNESS MEDITATION

Now let's learn about loving-kindness meditation. As mentioned earlier in the chapter, this is the meditation that was used to enhance self-transcendence, purpose in life, and DNA repair. There are different forms of this meditation, but here are the basics. Give it about twenty minutes, beginning just as you would with the breathing or mantra-based meditations:

- Find a comfortable place to sit, either in a chair or on the floor. Close your eyes. Take a few moments to just be, just *noticing* the sounds, smells, and feelings. Allowing yourself to settle down, turn your attention to your breathing.
- Notice the way your body automatically, effortlessly inhales and exhales.

- Don't try to manipulate your breath in any way. Notice the feeling of air moving in and out of the nose and the easy, natural way your body moves.

- Imagine yourself in a beautiful place. As you continue breathing in and out, say to yourself, "May I be happy and free of suffering." (You can use many other salutary phrases here such as "health" or "strength"—or create your own.)

- Next, imagine a new person entering your beautiful place. This is a person you care for a great deal. Again, as you continue breathing in and out, say to yourself, "May you be happy and free of suffering."

- Now move to another person entering your beautiful place. This is a person who provokes no feeling of like or dislike. A neutral person. It could be a bank teller or a waitress you recently interacted with. As you continue breathing in and out, say to yourself, "May you be happy and free of suffering."

- Now move to another person. A person who provokes feelings of dislike. Again, as you continue breathing in and out, say to yourself, "May you be happy and free of suffering."

- Finally, extend these feeling of loving-kindness to the world. To all living beings. Bring them into your special place and say to yourself, "May all beings be happy and free of suffering."

- Take a minute or so with your eyes shut before going
  back to your daily routine.

I really like the way this exercise is structured. It can be tough to extend, out of the blue, the same goodwill that I feel for my wife to the person who backed into her car in a parking lot last week, but working up to it in steps makes it considerably easier.

SIMPLE TIPS FOR INCREASING YOUR PRESENCE

Here are some simple techniques that you may want to try. Like the tips presented in each of the SPACE chapters, they're based on scientific knowledge and have been used successfully by real people.

- Come back to the moment by focusing on your breath. Inhale over a five-to-seven-second period, then exhale in over seven seconds. Start from your abdomen and let your chest fill up with air, like water filling a pitcher. Reverse the process on exhalation. Simple and effective.
- Our minds are generally in flit mode, rapidly shifting from one focus to another. It might have been a handy skill ten thousand years ago, but when did you last see a saber-toothed tiger? Take a moment to savor just one thing.
- Pick a tiny activity you do every day—putting on your

shoes, checking the weather, flossing—and let it fill up your whole consciousness. Then let it float away.

- Got half a minute? Grab it! Use it to center yourself. Those little in-between moments pop up throughout the day like unexpected gifts. Snag a few just for you. Bolster your mental presence (and resilience) with thirty seconds of mindful breathing (seven in, seven out) whenever the opportunity arises.

- Ever meditate at mealtime? Try this: Before your first bite, clear your mind. Then really savor the experience the way chefs and wine tasters do. Fully engage all your senses—taste, smell, touch, feel, sound—and take note of every detail.

- Do you normally flop into bed and doze off? Tonight, spend an extra fifteen minutes first, sitting (not lying) comfortably. Slow, deep breaths. Take in the silence, the darkness. Focus on how your body feels. Savor the moment. Let past and future dissolve into nothingness. Then hit the pillow.

- As kids, we used to take "penny hikes," letting a coin toss determine our direction at every crossroads or fork. We loved not knowing where we'd end up. Skip the coin; embrace the randomness. Simply take a walk with no destination, plan, or agenda and see where it leads you. Discover someplace new right around the corner.

- Feeling judgmental? Try a little forgiveness. Instead of

mentally taking others to task, try stepping into their shoes, their point of view. See if you can discover reasons behind their actions that might give you a deeper understanding of their situation. It's easy to be critical and defensive, but being consistently kind and empathetic is a much more certain and direct path to a self-transcending purpose, DNA repair, better health, and better relationships.

- Here's a weird one. If your mind keeps wandering, pretend for a moment that gravity has just gotten three times stronger. It's literally gluing your shoes to the floor—a perfect opportunity to focus on the here and now. Sometimes getting physically grounded works wonders in focusing your mind as well. Give it a try.

- Finding something (or someone) to blame is easy. They're everywhere, right? To change things up, try looking for reasons to be grateful instead. Take a moment, right now, and compose a brief "mental thank-you note" to a friend, author, plumber—whatever—who makes your life a little better. Got time? Send a real one right now.

- Poets and philosophers point out that we can't live in the past or the future. The present is all we ever have. For many, the past can be about revisiting regrets and the future just one big, scary unknown—or pipe dream. Why not revel in all the actual possibilities that exist in the present moment?

- You know that delicious moment just before sleeping or waking when kooky, random thoughts and images come swooping in? See if you can recapture that sense while you're awake. Take ten slow breaths, let go of all intention, then throw open your mind to anything that occurs to you.

- Walk like you mean it. Not fast, not slow, but steady and straight. Feel the ground under your feet. Listen to the rhythm of your steps, and pay attention to how it interacts with the rhythm of your breath. Enjoy being in motion.

- Take an analog holiday from your digital life—a "screen fast"—once in a while, maybe even once a day. Kind of like trading in a space heater for a fireplace.

- Athletes train by lifting weights, musicians by playing scales. Train your mind to be in the moment. Increase your presence by conscious observation. Spend a solid minute studying the simplest object at hand—a golf ball, a carrot, your left thumb—and describe every single detail that you can think of, without judgment.

- Finally, my SPECIAL SECRET MONKISH TIP: I don't allow myself an alcoholic beverage until I've meditated that day. Since I started this on January 1, 2014, I've never forgotten to meditate . . . though I sometimes forget to drink.

10

ACTIVITY

[We] praise the strong person, the good runner,
and each of the others because he naturally has
a certain character and is in a certain state in
relation to something good and excellent.

ARISTOTLE[1]

IF ARISTOTLE WERE ALIVE TODAY, HE'D VERY POSSIBLY BE A COACH. Or at least a sports fan. Given his many references to athletes, one could imagine that if his student, Alexander the Great, said, "Hey Aristotle, I've got two extra seats in my box for the races at the hippodrome tonight; wanna go? You can bring Plato." He'd put on his Team Athens toga and be completely down for it.

Aristotle valued habitual, strenuous physical exercise. He would have viewed a woman* like Aimee Mullins, the track and field star with prosthetic legs, as an exemplar of excellence (see chapter 6). If he were a coach, as classicist Kyle Oskvig suggests,[2] the sign in the locker room would read, "A good thing is better when it's more difficult."

Another standout on the Aristotelian Dream Team would be Mike Mosallam, who now, at thirty-six years old, is making it in the crazy world of Hollywood. He's head of production development for the largest independent television studio in the United States, where he works regu-

---

* Plato, Aristotle's mentor, publicly advocated the participation of women in sports.

larly with studio and production executives. That's just his day job—he also writes, directs, produces, and acts in his own films and television shows, including the acclaimed TLC series *All-American Muslim*.

"My purpose is to inspire," Mike told me. "I want to help people to live creatively and tell *their* story." He lives this purpose, but it takes everything he's got. "From the moment I wake up to the moment I go to bed, I have to be *on*. I don't ever get an opportunity to not be *on*, so to be my best self I have to be in great mental, physical, and spiritual shape."

I first met Mike over fifteen years ago, when he was a student in the University of Michigan's highly regarded musical theater program. Even then Mike was immensely talented, but he had one significant strike against him in the world of entertainment. At five feet seven inches and 265 pounds, he cut a wide figure. Food was an expression of culture in his Lebanese family, and Mike loved to, well . . . express his cultural heritage. But his heritage was also proving to be a burden.

As a result of the events of September 11, 2001, combined with growing awareness that he was gay in a traditional Muslim family, Mike went into the closet—actually, more like bank vault—and his weight became his "armor." "The one hundred extra pounds I was carrying around protected me from facing my fears."

Mike's "boat" had strong wind in the sails, but no rudder to steer—energy, but no willpower. "I don't think I had the capacity to even *have* willpower until I shed the armor," he says. He did it with "no pill, no surgery, no nothing. For the first twenty pounds I lost I only retrained how I eat. After that I started cardio training [treadmill]. Then got a personal trainer for the next forty pounds."

With every pound he dropped, Mike gathered more energy and willpower—sort of like a snowball in reverse that gets smaller as it accelerates up a hill. "There was a thrill in going from one level to another. I started running, hiking, rock climbing. Each time I could do a physical activity it became a thrill rush. I then ran my first half marathon. I'd never run for fun. I thought I'd only run when people were chasing me with some sort of weapon!"

This year a movie that he wrote, directed, and produced is going through the film festival circuit. He went on the pilgrimage (hajj) to Mecca. And he came out to his parents. Mike views each of these events as part of a process, a journey.

"My purpose is not something that I'll ever fully attain—it's a lifestyle—to live in a way that my actions are in line with this purpose." And physical activity is now an essential part of Mike's lifestyle.

WHAT IS PHYSICAL ACTIVITY?

The American College of Sports Medicine defines physical activity as "any bodily movement that is produced by the contraction of skeletal muscles and that substantially increases energy expenditure." Within this broad definition is exercise, which typically involves planned, structured, and repetitive body movement. This chapter is about physical activity in all aspects of daily living but it may be helpful to consider activities that can be "planned" and "structured."

Seemingly thousands of new exercise books are published each year, and I don't intend to add to the clutter of bewildering (and often contradictory) advice they offer. Instead, let's simplify things, starting with four types of exercise: aerobic, resistance, flexibility, and balance.

Aerobic: This type of exercise is also called "cardio," because it makes your lungs and heart move harder and faster. It's often divided into different levels of intensity and done for at least ten minutes at a time.[3] Examples of high-intensity aerobic activity are jogging or running, swimming laps, riding a bike fast or on hills, and playing singles tennis. Moderate-intensity aerobic activity includes walking fast, water aerobics, riding a bike on level ground, or playing doubles tennis.

Resistance: This is the kind of exercise that strengthens your muscles; it involves lifting weights, working with resistance bands, doing push-ups or sit-ups, and so forth. Your heart and breathing rates may increase, too, but that isn't the point of resistance training—increasing strength is. It isn't far from Aristotle's 2,300-year-old version of physical strength training, which developed, in his words, "the power of moving another thing as one wishes; and to move another thing, one must either pull, push, lift up, press down, or squeeze."[4]

Flexibility: These include range-of-motion activities such as neck, shoulder, upper body, chest, back, and other stretches. (Yoga, mentioned in the previous chapter, is a terrific way to get more flexible.)

Balance: These exercises, which focus on the way your brain and muscles work together, include balance, agility, coordination, and gait. Yoga, qigong, and tai chi all improve these skills.

All four of these categories of exercise are associated with improved health and energy,[5] and *many* government and health organizations have created their own specific guidelines. You can find and select recommendations from websites of the Centers for Disease Control and Prevention, the American College of Sports Medicine, the U.S. Surgeon General, and the Institute of Medicine, among others.

Shedding excess body fat, as Mike Mosallam did, is often best done through resistance training.[6] It's also been shown to build muscular strength and bone density. Not into lifting heavy weights? You're in luck. Recent research finds that high-repetition, light-resistance activity (working out with dumbbells or other weight equipment, for example) also increases muscle strength and bone density.

A good way to become more physically active is with a mix of moderate-to-vigorous aerobic and resistance training, stretching, and balancing exercises. Sure, really fit people generally get most of their activity through structured exercise.[7] But this doesn't mean that you can't get plenty of exercise in daily life. Walk your dog, bike to work, take the stairs instead of the elevator, walk to the airport gate rather than taking a tram or moving walkway. Yard work such as mowing, raking, gardening, and shoveling is terrific; so is housework like vacuuming, ironing, or making beds. (For that matter, so is some occupational work—how many obese mail carriers have you seen?)

I'm *not* going to recommend a particular type or level of activity for you. Everyone's different, both in what they can and are willing to do. But as a basic principle, start with things you like, and as your physical condition improves, you just might find yourself disliking the other things less.

If you have questions about whether certain types or levels of physical activity are right for you, ask your health-care professional. And if you've been physically inactive for some time or have a disability, it's definitely best to talk with your health-care professional before starting or changing an exercise routine.

It should go without saying that if you're a couch spud, *start slow.* At this very moment, the world's ER waiting rooms are packed with regular guys (and yes, it's mostly guys) who got a sudden urge to do a handspring or try to match their high school time in the hundred-yard dash. Worse, they're facing even more time as couch spuds, waiting for their sprains and strains to heal. This is nothing new. As Aristotle said, "Both excessive and defective exercise destroys the strength."

Mike Mosallam's story illustrates his gradually increasing ability to take on more physical activity, which in turn gave him greater energy and willpower. But not everybody is like Mike, so you'll need to select the right types and levels of activity that work for you.

If you don't know what those are, a good place to start is the U.S. Department of Health and Human Services' *Be Active Your Way: A Guide for Adults.*[8] It's easy to find on the Web, simple to follow, and was written by experts.

It's possible to adhere to most groups' activity recommendations yet still spend twenty-three and a half hours a day sitting or lying down. Are you an "active couch potato," who has active spurts but spends the rest of the day on their rump? Researchers have found in numerous studies that this kind of sedentary behavior has negative effects on disease, hospitalization, and death, *independent* of physical activity.[9] In other words, increased hours of television watching reduces energy during the day and physical activity alone doesn't make up for it.

THE WHY

People get more active for many reasons. For some it's weight loss. For others it's to manage stress, or for better health (used in the traditional medical sense of "absence of disease"). It might also be for increased well-being (which is the eudaimonic and, I believe, more accurate definition of health). Michelle Segar and her colleagues at the University of Michigan asked women to give their most important reasons for getting active.[10] Since physical activity is all about participation, Michelle wanted to learn which reasons were the most, and least, motivating.

Michelle's research showed that the most commonly cited reasons for physical activity were "losing weight" and "better health." "Well-being" was cited *least*. Interestingly, though, the women listing well-being as their top physical activity goal had over 30 percent *more* participation than those with weight-loss or health goals.

Why is that?

As Segar explains in her book, *No Sweat,* the "the foundation of sustainable behavior change" for physical activity is not the *how,* but the *why.* In a separate study,[11] Segar and her colleagues found that losing weight and improved health were not "intrinsic," but "controlling" reasons for physical activity. Women giving those reasons felt that they *should* be more active and felt guilty if they didn't exercise.

The intrinsic motivator of well-being, on the other hand, was indeed more motivating.

NO PLEASURE, NO GAIN

Aristotle never said that hedonic pleasure was a bad thing; he just warned us about getting so much of it that we start tuning out our inner self (our daimon). Pleasure is . . . well, pleasurable. And no matter how much energy and willpower physical activity brings us, without joy it can be tough to stick with the program.

So make sure you do things you like, or at least do them in a setting that you enjoy. I walk to work nearly every day and can listen to books on my smartphone. It's a special time to learn something new. Mike Mosallam told me that he didn't necessarily enjoy lifting weights, but at least there were "all these cute guys" at his gym. In other words, the road to purpose can be paved with pleasure.

A NOT-SO-SIMPLE ACTIVITY TIP

Physical environments shape physical activity. If there are stairs where you work, are they dim and ugly (or worse, unsafe) or attractive and brightly lit? Is there space for an exercise or yoga class? (Fun fact: a typical yoga mat only takes up twelve square feet!) You might ask the boss if you can use a stand-up desk or table. We have some at JOOL Health, and they're *always full*.

What's good for the workplace is good for the community. Don't neglect your neighborhood. If you're not lucky enough to live close to open spaces, parks, and trails, do whatever you can to advocate for them. Sometimes when I travel I find myself judging people for staying cooped up in their cars instead of walking . . . until I notice that there are no safe sidewalks or shade trees. A community garden, public basketball or tennis courts, bike paths, speed bumps, marked crosswalks, and curb-cuts all make your neighborhood a better place to be active and have more fun, all while watching your property value tick up. Bring us some shrubbery!

SIMPLE ACTIVITY TIPS

Like the ones presented in the other SPACE chapters, these tips are based on scientific knowledge and have been used successfully by real people.

- Don't tell my television producer friend Mike Mosallam's boss, but Mike feels we should all be watching less TV—or at least thinking more about how we watch. "I watch certain shows," he tells me. "I DVR [record] almost everything and rarely watch things in real time." He also says we should also be more selective about what we watch: "With the oversaturation of content these days, it may take a little more effort to find, but TV can be a fun workout for your mind. Sheesh, trying to keep up with who's who on *Game of Thrones* must definitely burn some calories!"

- Speaking of video, instead of exercising just one finger—the one on your remote's fast-forward button—let the ads play out while you get up and move your whole body. Hit the mute button and spend five minutes showing your body you care. Even a few push-ups, jumping jacks, and squats can add up fast.

- That thirty-minute phone call with a relative or close friend? If they're local, join them for a hike instead. Turn all that family reminiscing into more than just a stroll down memory lane: walk faster around the local park, or climb a hill when talk turns to juicy gossip. And if they're not local? Well, the cell phone may have turned us all into glassy-eyed zombies, but it also provides invaluable opportunities to *move*. Lace up your shoes and start walking while talking.

- Park from the shopping mall or grocery store so you can snag a few extra steps. How about taking the longest distance between two points once in while?

- Shake things up at the office by scheduling your next meeting on the hoof. Take your colleagues around the corner for a brisk saunter in the fresh air. The exercise will increase blood flow, distributing more oxygen throughout the body, including your brain.

- Treat your workout the same as you'd treat an appointment with your boss or your doctor. Put it on your calendar and *commit* to it, no matter how much you have going on or how much you'd rather stretch out on the couch for a leisurely nap. Committing to exercise can make it happen.

- Give your kaffeeklatsch the hotfoot. Next time you meet a friend for coffee, ask for a to-go cup and get in some extra steps. Movement can actually stimulate conversation. Vitamin D from the sun, a little caffeine, and a brisk saunter around town.

- Make a micro-investment in an activity tracker (I just found one online for ninety-five cents) and start counting your steps. There are plenty of monitoring apps for smartphones, too. Some phones even come with built-in pedometers. Start with a not-too-challenging goal (maybe 7,500 steps a day), then slowly increase it.

- Monitoring can be motivating: "I'll hit ten thousand steps today with one more quick stroll after dinner." The benefits of increased energy, improved sleep, resilience, and stamina often show up quickly with consistent effort.

- Have a "standing" date with yourself. If you have a sedentary job (or if you're just a sedentary person), set the alarm on your watch or phone to go off every hour during the day, and whenever it goes off, get up for five minutes for a stretch or a brisk walk. It's a snooze button in reverse: a great way to reset both your body and your brain.

- Go ahead—be "that person." The one who takes the stairs instead of the elevator. Just a few steps can burn calories. Do that a few times each day and watch your stamina take flight, too.

- Now that you've become "that person," be "that person" in the kitchen, too. Meal prep can be a bit boring at times . . . why not toss some up-tempo music into the mix? This recipe calls for some extra spice. Salsa, polka, Beyoncé. Shake it up a little while you move about the kitchen. Just make sure to put the knife down first.

- Get active and do some good at the same time. Join a fund-raising walk/run or do a 5K for a cause you want to lend your support to. Or help build a house for the homeless, collect trash, or clean up a park. Self-transcending physical activity is a great way to get more energy.

- If you can't walk all the way to work because of distance, terrain, or weather, maybe you can still walk *part* of the way. Pick a parking spot, or a bus or subway stop, that's not necessarily the closest one, and you'll get the blood circulating at the beginning or end of your work day.

- You don't need to get all of your exercise in at one time. Try squeezing in a few ten-minute intervals when you have time.

- Take a friendship to the next level. Become workout pals. Having a workout compadre can be motivating and keep you accountable, as well as bring a whole new dimension to your friendship.
- Next time you're walking somewhere, pick up the pace a little. Turn it into your own little Jedi mind trick: pretend you have somewhere really important to be and you're running late.
- As anyone who's taken a long flight in a cramped seat knows, holding still can be a lot more tiring than moving. The same holds true with desks and couches: after a day of zero activity, you may feel exhausted, but you can quickly turn things around with a brief burst of action.

This chapter covered some of the basics of activity but emphasized the need for a personal, choice-driven plan. The "why" is more important than the "how." Then, selecting activities that you enjoy is a good next step. Creating your own approach to physical activity is fun.

In fact, it's fun to create just about anything! Let's turn to that next.

11

CREATIVITY

Here, when the danger to his will is greatest, art
approaches as a saving sorceress, expert at healing.

FRIEDRICH NIETZSCHE[1]

CONSIDER A BRICK (REAL OR IMAGINED). WRITE DOWN ALL THE things you could do with it (to keep things civil, let's exclude the obvious use as a weapon to bonk someone on the head with).

A doorstop? Good! A paperweight? Fine! When giving workshops on creativity, I generally receive five to eight perfectly good uses for a brick. But in Omaha, Nebraska, a group of architects in my workshop came up with thirty-seven. One person suggested grinding up the brick to make pigment for painting or cosmetics. Another came up with a novel and extraordinarily bizarre sex toy, which I won't describe here.

Psychologists use this brick exercise, among other strategies, to measure creativity. Specifically, they look for the number—and novelty—of uses for a brick. Midwestern architects are clearly off the charts. How about you? How many did you come up with?

Do you consider yourself a creative person? How creative were you last year? How about during the past twenty-four hours? Only 52 percent of Americans describe themselves as creative, and fewer than 40 percent feel that they're living up to their creative potential. Of the sleep, presence, activity, creativity, and eating (SPACE) behaviors, we've found daily, self-reported ratings of creativity to be, by far, the lowest. On a scale of one (low) to five (high), the average rating is a two.

What has society done to us? Or put another way, what have we done to ourselves? If you ask a classroom of second graders if they're creative, nearly all hands would reach for the sky (even mine, rising Iwo Jima–like from the teacher's trash can). How do we get back the creative energy we once had as children?

Edward Hirsch, poet and author of *How to Read a Poem,*[2] says, "There's never been a culture without art. Never been a culture without poetry. Never been a culture without music. They must be delivering something to us that we really need for our psyches."[3] I frankly find it difficult to understand why we let the creative arts play such a minor role in our children's education, let alone in our adult lives.

Hirsch and others collaborate with my friend Jeremy Nobel, a physician at Harvard's medical school and founder of the Foundation for Art and Healing. The foundation works with veterans and patients, among other groups, to promote healing through creating, sharing, and receiving art. Does it work? You bet. Studies have demonstrated the efficacy of artistic expression on immune system improvement and reduction of stress, fatigue, and pain.[4] These studies have been done on many age groups and with different types of illness, from PTSD to cancer. Researchers are still trying to understand the reasons that the arts have such an impact on health and well-being, but *emotional expression* is clearly an important piece of the puzzle.

In a nationwide study that started in 1996,[5] over seven hundred

Americans were asked about the degree to which they expressed their emotions. Twelve years later, those who reported high levels of emotional expression were living over three years longer and were far less likely to suffer cancer or heart disease than those with lower levels of expression.

APPRECIATION

Creative activities allow us to express our emotions and become more vital. And not just when we're the ones doing the painting, writing, dancing, or singing, but also when we're the ones doing the *appreciating*. In the Swedish study described in chapter 6, the researchers found positive effects on both physical and mental health not only from choral singing (creating) but also from watching a film, going to an art museum, or listening to a concert (appreciating).[6]

Creating and *appreciating* something may seem like two very different activities, but the psychologist Rollo May suggests that they spark a similar process:

> When we engage a painting . . . we are experiencing some new moment of sensibility. Some new vision is triggered in us by our contact with the painting; something unique is born in us. This is why appreciation of the music or painting or other works of the creative person is also a creative act on our part.[7]

Of course, the art that we appreciate can be happy art (like Pharrell Williams's 2014 hit song, "Happy") or it can be sad or tragic art (like Bernstein and Sondheim's "Somewhere" from the musical *West Side Story*). Aristotle observed that sad art, such as a tragic play, is cathartic, providing an emotional release and cleansing. As for music, he said, "All experience a certain purge and pleasant relief . . . cathartic melodies give innocent joy to men."[8]

Was Aristotle right? Do we get "innocent joy" from sad music? If we're feeling blue, wouldn't upbeat party music be better for us than the blues? Research evidence suggests that Aristotle's observations still hold true today: sad music evokes a pleasurable, cathartic release.[9] In fact, sad music creates *pleasurable* emotions whether or not the listener is sad to begin with.[10] This seems odd, because sad music activates regions of the brain associated with sadness. What's going on?

The emotions that we tend to feel when listening to sad music include peacefulness, tenderness, nostalgia (since so many sad songs evoke specific memories), and even self-transcendence.[11] We feel empathy, for . . . whom? The composer? The performer? Humanity itself?

It's my view that sad art makes us feel more connected, both with the artist and with our fellow man, and that even sad emotions can be pleasurable. Not pleasure in the hedonic sense. Shakespeare's *Romeo and Juliet,* Edvard Munch's *The Scream,* Alvin Ailey's *Cry,* or Maurice Ravel's *Pavane for a Dead Princess* certainly don't evoke feelings of being at Disney World (unless you're in a long line), but they do allow us to share such human experiences as tragedy, loss, or chaos . . . followed by an existential group hug.

Friedrich Nietzsche points out that tragic art, rather than depressing us, can be uplifting and transforming. In *Twilight of the*

Idols, Nietzsche writes, "The tragic artist is not a pessimist—it is precisely he who affirms all that is questionable and terrible in existence, he is Dionysian."*

An example is the movie *Melancholia,* which deals with (spoiler alert) the end of the world. As former *Los Angeles Times* film critic Betsy Sharkey put it, "How does the world end? When it is in the hands of the cinematic master of human misery, dark Danish auteur Lars von Trier, as it is in *Melancholia,* it ends in extraordinary, horrific, searing, aching and unthinkable ways. It is his most hopeful film yet."[12]

So to develop your own creativity, you may want to consider getting out and appreciating the arts. Perhaps even a deep, sad movie that doesn't involve comic-book heroes.

CREATIVITY IN EVERYDAY LIFE

Creative expression is not only found in traditional arts such as movies, music, painting, writing, poetry, dance, and theater. In fact, an important step toward becoming more creative is to observe and take part in the creativity that can be found in daily life.

Researchers talk about two essential elements of a creative endeavor: novelty and usefulness. A custodian may come up with a new schedule for waxing floors in an office building (novel) that results in easier access for employees (useful). A teacher may concoct a new lesson

---

* Dionysus was the Greek god of wine and of joy and freedom. Also known as Bacchus.

plan for teaching (novel) that results in higher student performance (useful). A couple may improvise a kinky new sex game involving a brick (novel) that results in a stronger relationship (useful). These innovators may not even think of themselves as "creative"—but they are.

My main high school interest, science, led me to the standard geeky clubs and activities—chess, computers, beekeeping—that left little time for the arts. I certainly didn't think of myself as "creative." Not until college, that is, when I met Jeri, an artist and my future wife. In contrast to my own self-image, she thought that I had a creative side and helped me find ways to bring that part of me into the science-ish things I did.

Creativity is now among the attributes that I value most dearly in my career and life. Not only does it give me more energy, it's also a central requirement for staying aligned with my purpose.

PURPOSE

Harvard professor David Perkins suggests that, whether designing a thumbtack or a heat shield for a spacecraft, the creative process starts not with a theoretical concept but with a purpose: in these two cases, to attach paper to the wall or to keep astronauts from burning up on reentry. The necessities inherent in purposeful living also stimulate creative solutions. A parent with a demanding job must be innovative to successfully balance work and family. An older person with a physical disability must find creative solutions in order to care for a loved one.

Necessity is the mother of invention, and purpose is the mother of necessity.

My own goal of helping others find greater purpose brings with it "necessities" requiring creative solutions. How to reach millions of people? In the past, Viktor Frankl, who had a similar purpose in life, wrote an incredible book (*Man's Search for Meaning*) and created a powerful new form of therapy (logotherapy). My response to the same need over half a century later was to create a graphic novel and accompanying app (*On Purpose*), then this book (*Life on Purpose*), and then, using the engine of modern entrepreneurism, a daily-use app for purposeful living (JOOL Health).

"A FOOL RUSHING AHEAD"

Author Monte Montgomery wrote a children's book with his wife, Claire, called *Hubert Invents the Wheel*.[13] In ancient Mesopotamia, teenaged inventor Hubert grows weary of dragging rocks and other heavy objects on a flat sledge, so he comes up with the wheel. Society's reception of his creative solution, like the reception to many innovations, is not positive. Rather than being hailed as a hero, Hubert is regarded as lazy and simply trying to get out of work. His real struggle wasn't creating the wheel but getting society to accept it.

A similar point is made in Douglas Adams's *Hitchhiker's Guide to the Galaxy*,[14] when the earth sends an unsuspecting group—all of the hairdressers and marketers in the world, among others—to a different planet. Starting a new civilization is tough; it takes years to complete the "difficult" invention of the wheel. The protagonist Ford Prefect asks,

> "Difficulty? What do you mean, difficulty? It's the single simplest machine in the entire Universe!"
> The marketing girl soured him with a look. "All right, Mr. Wiseguy," she said, "if you're so clever, you tell us what *color* it should be."

People might find this fictional comment ridiculous, which it of course is, but real-life creative thinkers are used to icy blasts from the status quo. Some examples:[15]

- The radio had "no imaginable commercial value" as a device that sends "a message to nobody in particular" (from investors).
- Pasteur's germ theory was "ridiculous fiction" (from a famous professor of physiology, 1872).
- The telephone had "too many shortcomings" and had "no value to us" (Western Union, 1876). In other words, "Everything that can be invented has been invented" (commissioner of the U.S. Patent and Trademark Office, 1899).

A few more howlers: The Barbie Doll was "too adult."[16] The Beatles played "guitar music" that was "on the way out."[17] Dr. Seuss's first book was "too different."[18] Anne Frank's *Diary of a Young Girl* was "dreary."[19] And my personal favorite? *The Great Gatsby* would be decent if F. Scott Fitzgerald would only "get rid of that Gatsby character."[20]

In my own laboratory we spent over a decade demonstrating the significant impact of deeply tailored, computer-generated programs to help people quit smoking, change their diet, and prevent cancer. The interventions were easy to use and could be delivered inexpensively to millions of people, and their efficacy rate rivaled that of cost- and labor-intensive human counseling.

When we offered our software to the U.S. Centers for Disease Control (CDC), my colleagues and I were told that *"people won't use the Internet for their health."* After this rejection, I feared that my research would have a distressingly low impact: I'd go to my grave with the number of journal articles on my headstone instead of the number of people I'd helped. So in 1998 I created HealthMedia, Inc., an Internet-based health coaching company, which has reached over fifty million people: innovation generated by necessity generated by a purpose.

Rollo May said that creativity requires courage and that courage is needed in every profession if one is to innovate and progress. But innovation is a *subversive* activity—an act that entails a deliberate disruption of the status quo. The nineteenth-century French painter Edgar Degas wrote that "[a] painter paints a picture with the same feeling as that with which a criminal commits a crime."[21]

With such disruption often comes enmity and alienation from the status quo. You sense this in the memoir of the Swiss psychiatrist

Carl Jung as he describes the toll taken by his "daimon of creativity": "There was a daimon in me, and in the end its presence proved decisive . . . I had to hasten on, to catch up with my vision. Since my contemporaries, understandably, could not perceive my vision, they saw only a fool rushing ahead."[22]

Creativity isn't for the faint of heart. Carl Jung's understanding of, and connection to, his inner self (his daimon) produced great turbulence in his personal life. This is bound to happen when one creates a new form of psychotherapy that flaunts the prevailing egos (Sigmund Freud's in particular). Having enrolled in the Nietzschean "how to slay your 'thou shalt' dragon" school, Jung—like many artists, innovators, and entrepreneurs—found himself at odds with many of his colleagues. He was willing to live with this.

Jung uses the word *individuation* to describe the emergence of the inner self: "it is the process by which individual beings are formed and differentiated . . . it is the development of the psychological individual as being distinct from the general, collective psychology."[23] Individuation is a popular theme among artists, since it's associated with the development of one's creative style.

STYLE

Nietzsche said, "One thing is needful. To 'give style' to one's character—a great and rare art! It is practiced by those who survey all the strengths and weaknesses of their nature and then fit them into an artistic plan until every one of them appears as art and reason and even weaknesses delight the eye."[24] (See what I mean? Even his defense of style is stylish!)

Perhaps inevitably, scientists have even quantified and analyzed artistic style. For example, William Shakespeare tended to use particular words (such as the noun *will*) with a different frequency in his plays than did Ben Jonson, Thomas Middleton, or John Fletcher.[25] Each author has a common vocabulary from which to draw words, but each author makes an individual selection from this vocabulary, thus creating their own style.

In life we don't each have the same "vocabulary" of options to draw from. Donald Trump, for example, can select a private jet from his vocabulary while most of us cannot. There are, however, many elements in life from which we can select and create our individual style. We often admire people who've been able to move beyond the "general, collective psychology," as Jung put it, to create a style that reflects their inner self.

I'm sure you have your own list, but when I think of individuals like Michelle Obama, Steve Jobs, Arianna Huffington, Richard Branson, Eleanor Roosevelt, Winston Churchill, and hundreds of other individuals with very purposeful lives, I think of the style they had— not just what they did, but *how* they did it. And, as Nietzsche adds, "In the end, when the work is finished, it becomes evident how the constraint of a single taste governed and formed everything large and small. Whether this taste was good or bad is less important than one might suppose, if only it was a single taste!"[26]

Nietzsche, of course, wasn't talking about private jets, glamorous clothes, or a new hairdo (though he did have a killer mustache) but about the process of creating an authentic, unified self despite the massive influences of society to not be yourself.

BRICKS AND BRAINS

Let's return to the "What can you do with a brick?" exercise. In studying how people create new, useful concepts, scientists have generally moved away from the view that creativity is a single concept. Neuroscientists, in fact, are finding complex increases and decreases in activity of various brain regions during the act of creation.

A consistent finding from brain studies is that during the generative phase of creation—whether jazz improvisation, rap music, or poetry—a part of the brain associated with the self (the medial prefrontal cortex, or mPFC) becomes engaged while we disengage from the self-*controlling* and inhibitory function of our brain (associated with the dorsolateral prefrontal cortex, or dlPFC). During an editing or evaluative phase of the creative process, researchers find that the control function reengages. In fact, one study found that expert poets had greater reduction of the self-controlling function than novices and that the quality of poetry created during the study was associated with these brain functions.[27]

These findings are supported by studies of different forms of meditation.[28] The focused meditation (for example, focusing on the breath or a mantra) discussed in chapter 9 has been found to enhance self-control but can also reduce creativity whereas observational meditation (being more present and aware of immediate sensations and stimuli) reduces inhibition and increases creativity. Over dinner in his home city of Amsterdam, the senior researcher of this research, Matthijs Baas, predicted a time in the near future when we should be able to prescribe the right type of mindfulness practice based on what we were doing that day (for example, generating versus editing new creations).

So we can imagine that, while thinking of various uses for a brick, we become highly engaged in the exercise while reducing our inhibitions regarding what a brick should be. With inhibition reduced, we can consider unusual or novel properties of the brick—for example, not only its size and weight, but also its shape, texture, color, smell, taste, density, sound when struck, chemical makeup, suitability as a hat, and so forth. Creativity demands that we expand the concept of a brick beyond the usual attributes of "brickiness." Then, as we evaluate the usefulness of the ideas we generated, our self-control processes reengage, moving back and forth between generation and evaluation, until we're the proud possessors of a novel, useful function for the brick.

Creative people must be able to divorce themselves from known associations of the concept. Telling ourselves that we *can* indeed grind the brick into powder to make paint requires an ability we spoke of earlier—to flout the status quo. I have a sense that really great designers lap the field in this ability: they don't seem to let generally accepted standards get in their way. Frank Gehry, love him or hate him, is a case in point.

Speaking of designers, Michael Graves was a leading American architect, designing noteworthy buildings around the world. At the age of sixty-eight a spinal cord infection paralyzed him from the waist down, and he found himself spending a lot of time in the hospital. He told Thomas Goetz at a WIRED Health conference that he was tired of the way the tray on his over-bed hospital table bumped into his stomach, so he worked with Stryker, the hospital furniture company, to completely redesign the table.

Graves didn't stop there. Frustrated with the wheelchair he was given (mPFC is engaged), he and his firm began designing wheelchairs. He became, in his own words, a "reluctant healthcare expert" but did so with no inhibitions (dlPFC is disengaged) regarding the way wheelchairs should be designed. He then went on to design better equipment, furniture, and even hospitals themselves.

Most people in hospital rooms are trying to recover, not complaining about the furniture. They wouldn't be courageous enough to say, "Thanks for taking care of me, but your furniture is horrible!" Michael Graves directly experienced illness (becoming the mPFC-engaged Nietzschean camel), then questioned the status quo (the dlPFC disengaged lion), then created a new response to the status quo (the mPFC-engaged and dlPFC-disengaged child).

His innovations were driven by necessity, which was driven by purpose. Graves puts it even more succinctly: "I want to do as much healthcare as I can before I croak."[29] Again, why is it that we have to be near death before finding a great purpose? If you'd like to increase your creativity before you croak, here are some ideas.

SIMPLE TIPS FOR INCREASING YOUR CREATIVITY

Like the tips presented in the other SPACE chapters, these are based on scientific knowledge and have been used successfully by real people.

- Get empathic. We don't need to get as sick as Michael Graves to become the Nietzschean camel, but we do need to become empathic. In her book *inGenius,* Stanford University educator Tina Seelig writes, "When you empathize, you are, essentially, changing your frame of reference by shifting your perspective to that of the other person."

- Spend a few bucks on a sketchbook and some art pencils; then get busy. With even a few minutes of practice a day, you'll be amazed at how fast you improve—not just at drawing, but at observing.

- The blues aren't necessarily a bad thing. University of British Columbia researchers found that keeping the color blue in sight stimulates creativity. Paint a wall. Change your screen saver. Buy a poster. Turn your nails periwinkle. Splash some blue around.

- Stuck on a problem? Step outside your head for a minute. How might your best friend approach the same problem? A scientist? A poet? A six-year-old? Your dog? A fresh solution—even a hilariously wrong one—might lead to a right one.

- Learning a new skill can give a big boost to the ones

you already have. In most communities you can find fun classes in everything from aerobics to zither. Surround yourself with enthusiastic beginners just like you.

- Mentally frozen? Thaw yourself out with physical movement. Take a walk. Mail a letter. Buy milk. Stretch. Maybe it wasn't the falling apple that inspired Isaac Newton's theory of gravity; maybe it was the stroll to the orchard. Einstein is said to have come up with $E = mc^2$ while taking a walk.

- Play: it's not just for kids anymore. If there's room on your desk for a coffee cup and a sandwich, there's room for a Slinky, some blocks, and a windup dinosaur. Childhood was often our most creative period; then adults took our toys away. Take them back.

- Clear the clutter. It's easy to spot one (or twenty) little daily annoyances that trip you up, slow you down, or block your view of the Big Picture. This is also a great way to improve willpower.

- Reality programs are popular because they show us the world through the eyes of crab fishermen, master chefs, storm chasers, and so forth. But guess what: every day we're surrounded by real people—in real life—who are totally different from us! Spend some time with them; it'll broaden your horizons and theirs.

- Remember those goofy collages we made in school? Turns out they're a great way to use images and spatial relationships to unravel grown-up problems. All you need is a stack of old magazines, a cork or poster board, and your imagination. Tip: keep your collage someplace visible so it stays fresh in your mind.

- Because we use language to write, speak, and think, it can either imprison or free us. Use a dictionary or "word a day" website to keep expanding your vocabulary—your creativity will expand right along with it. Anyone interested in a "dulcet" evening swim at the lake tonight?

- Researchers have long known that smell, more than any other sense, triggers emotion and memory. It can unlock creativity, too. Rosemary, cinnamon, and vanilla scents have been shown to help test subjects concentrate and create. Find out what works for you. Have fun exploring some new smells, herbs, spices, or fragrances.

- Random, cheap creativity boosters: buy two-for-one play tickets; cook with an ingredient you never use (kale tastes better than it smells); buy a used ukulele; take at least one beginning yoga class (even if you don't like yoga, you'll meet interesting, attractive people).

- In the movie *My Dinner with Andre,* Andre tells Wally to "do everything left-handed for a day, to break the habit." This sounds dangerous, but there are other ways to switch things up: find a new radio station; read the first chapter of a book you expect to hate; surprise an old friend with a phone call. In short, keep it fresh.

- Adults worry; children create. Spend some time around young people and try to figure out *how they do that*. If they're yours, do something that they (not you) suggest. If they're someone else's, just go with the flow. Pretend you're on a safari of observation and understanding: "Who are these strange homunculi, and why are they so alive?"

- Creativity's a little like playing right field: long periods of tense waiting, punctuated by bursts of frenzied action. If nothing's come your way for a while, leave the ballpark. Jump into something completely different. You'll come back later, refreshed and ready to snag a whole bunch of fresh ideas coming your way.

By the way, here's another great use for a brick (or several). Fire up your grill. Flatten a whole chicken by pushing hard on the breast-bone; then rub it with olive oil. Season with salt and pepper. Place the chicken on the grill, skin side down, over indirect heat, setting *bricks* on top, and grill until skin is golden and crisp, twenty-five to thirty minutes. Using tongs (sturdy ones!), remove the bricks and turn the chicken skin-side up. Replace the bricks and continue grilling twenty-five to thirty minutes longer, or until the chicken is cooked through and an instant-read thermometer inserted into the thickest part of the thigh registers 165 degrees. Thank Saint Lawrence, patron saint of grilling, for the great meal.

Bon appétit! Which, by the way, brings us to the next chapter . . .

12

EATING

If you truly get in touch with a piece of carrot, you
get in touch with the soil, the rain, the sunshine.
You get in touch with Mother Earth and eating in
such a way, you feel in touch with true life, your
roots, and that is meditation. If we chew every
morsel of our food in that way we become grateful
and when you are grateful, you are happy.

THICH NHAT HANH[1]

IF YOU WERE A JUDGE LISTENING TO A PRISONER'S PLEA FOR PAROLE, what factors would influence your decision? The prisoner's number of previous incarcerations? The severity of the crime? The time already served? The availability of a rehabilitation program? Would you be influenced by the prisoner's age? Gender? Religion?

How about by a sandwich and some fruit?

In a 2002 study[2] conducted in Israel, judges were monitored minute by minute throughout the day to determine what factors influenced their parole decisions. Two of the main factors turned out to be the prisoners' previous incarcerations and the availability of a rehabilitation program.

The judges were *far* more influenced, however, by whether they'd just eaten a meal. In the morning, after breakfast, the judges granted parole to roughly 65 percent of the prisoners. As the morning wore on, the parole rate dropped to nearly zero. Then they would have a snack, and the parole rate went back to roughly 65 percent. As the early afternoon dragged on, the parole rate would drop to 10 percent. After a midafternoon lunch, it shot back up to around 65 percent again.

What, how much, and when we eat has a huge influence on the way we think and act. If we want more energy and willpower, we must eat well. This chapter cuts through all the fad diets, supplements, and super foods and has a simple goal: to help you *build a sustainable diet for daily energy and willpower*.

To reach this goal, it would be difficult to find a better starting point than the . . .

MEDITERRANEAN DIET

As with all of the SPACE practices, it helps to start with behaviors that you already enjoy. You're unlikely to sustain a diet without getting hedonic pleasure from it. After all, most of us love to eat. The Greeks and Italians may struggle with managing their economies, but they certainly know how to rustle up a plate of grub.

The Mediterranean diet has been shown in large research studies to be easy to adopt and sustain. Why? Because it tastes so amazingly good.

You can find out more about the Mediterranean diet along with wonderful recipes on the Web, but here are the basics. It doesn't just cover a plate with a giant hunk of meat; Mediterraneans are more likely to use meat as a flavor and texture, or simply to leave it out altogether. For example:

- Throw a little minced prosciutto into a simple but spicy tomato sauce, spoon it over al dente pasta, and pair it with some red wine. Or . . .
- Take a nice fish and broil or grill it with a squeeze of orange and serve it with vegetables and a crusty bread. Oh, and don't forget the white wine. Or . . .
- Or how about a quick lunch of bow tie pasta mixed with pesto and some fresh vegetables? Grate just a little Parmesan cheese (not a mountain) over the top. Or . . .
- Buy a whole chicken and try the brick chicken recipe at the end of the previous chapter; serve it with wild rice and a glass of—you guessed it—wine!

Poultry and fish figure prominently in the Mediterranean Diet, but if you're more adventurous, try rabbit or game birds. Red meat is used more as a flavorful condiment than as the centerpiece of a meal. Plant-based foods are regulars on the plate. Spices (ideally fresh ones) are essential, as is olive oil, for both cooking and bread dipping. As I said, wine is encouraged . . . in moderation. Butter is almost entirely absent, and so is refined sugar.

A word about sugar. Glucose is an essential part of our diet and is closely related to energy and willpower. To return to the study of the Israeli judges, Nobel Prize–winning researcher Daniel Kahneman told National Public Radio, "When you're depleted, you tend to fall back on default actions, and the default action in that case is apparently to deny parole. So yes, people are strongly influenced by the level of glucose in the brain."[3]

In the Mediterranean diet, glucose comes from the carbohydrates found in the vegetables, fruits, beans, nuts, bread, pasta, rice, couscous (try it!), potatoes, and yogurt. As we'll see, these are far better ways to deliver glucose to your body than by inhaling candy bars.

GLUCOSE IN THE BRAIN

The brain of the average adult human makes up about 2 percent of body weight but burns approximately 20 percent of our energy[4]— proportionally, greater than any other body part. And that energy comes from glucose.

We've mentioned brain activity quite a bit in this book, particularly as we've examined how various parts of the brain are used for different activities (such as meditating or thinking about purposeful values). This "activation" refers to the increased signaling of neurons, which requires energy. As you may have learned in biology class, the oxidation of glucose to carbon dioxide and water results in the production of large amounts of energy in the form of adenosine triphosphate (ATP).[5] In other words, no glucose, no energy. No energy, no brain activity.

GLUCOSE AND WILLPOWER

One such glucose-fueled brain activity (actually a set of activities) is self-control, or willpower. Hypoglycemia (low blood glucose) is associated with a lack of self-control. As mentioned earlier, the book *Will-power* by Roy Baumeister and John Tierney[6] reports that low glucose levels are found in over 90 percent of juvenile delinquents and that hypoglycemia is associated with traffic violations, public profanity, shoplifting, destruction of property, exhibitionism, public masturbation, embezzlement, arson, spouse abuse, and child abuse!

So will increasing gummy bear intake prevent us from smashing store windows and topping it off with a wank on Main Street? Thank goodness there's no study of this. But studies have demonstrated that sips of lemonade with sugar (glucose) versus lemonade with diet sweetener improves willpower.[7] This result supports findings in the general population that overweight and obese individuals drink more diet beverages than healthy-weight individuals and that, importantly, heavier people who drink diet beverages consume more solid-food calories than those who drink sugar-sweetened beverages.[8]

Note that I'm not recommending the excessive consumption of sugary soft drinks, which would give you *way* more glucose than you need. The best way to ensure a slow, steady release of glucose throughout the day is to eat foods that are low in what dietitians call "glycemic load." Not coincidentally, these tend to be the staples of the Mediterranean diet: vegetables and fruits, yogurt, multigrain breads and cereals, beans and chickpeas (hummus), and nuts.

High-glycemic-load foods (such as rice, pasta, and baked goods made with white flower) produce a sharp spike in blood glucose, which is usually followed by a sharp drop, resulting in fatigue and hunger. Conversely, eating low-glycemic-load foods through the day "smooths out the bumps," allowing you to maintain your energy and willpower without gorging on a huge lunch or dinner.

Are whole grains, such as whole wheat bread, really that much better for you? In his book *The Story of the Human Body,*[9] Harvard paleoanthropologist Daniel Lieberman points out that the outer bran and germ layers that surround the starchy part of the seed contain the large portion of healthy oils, vitamins, and minerals. Farmers long ago learned that they could store these food staples longer by removing the outer layer, leaving little pods of starch.

With modern storage methods, however, we can now readily serve, for example, brown rice, which has roughly the same caloric content as white rice but three to six times as much vitamin B and E, magnesium, potassium, and phosphorus. Brown rice also contains more fiber, contributing to our sense of fullness—we feel fuller sooner and are less likely to overeat.

Finally, it should be noted that while wine is encouraged in the Mediterranean diet, alcohol intake can decrease your blood glucose, resulting in less energy and willpower. This may be one explanation of why one drink of alcohol leads to another, which leads to another.

UP A NOTCH

Studies have shown that it's fairly easy to switch from giant plates of red meat to the Mediterranean diet. Among my own family, friends, and acquaintances, those who make the change usually love the new diet and don't look back. They also find it easier to lose weight than they did with low-fat or low-carbohydrate diets.[10]

The Mediterranean diet is largely plant based, so it's not a huge stretch to remove the meat entirely and, over time, become a vegetarian. A gradual approach helps, just as switching from whole milk to skim is easier if you go by way of 2 percent, then 1 percent. You might try other cuisine options as well—Indian, Thai, and Chinese cuisines have wonderful vegetarian options.

Want to take it up a notch? Actually a couple of notches? The vegans I know are super-healthy, and the data don't lie—switching from a meat to a vegan diet gives you more energy, is better for the planet, *and* is surprisingly easy to adopt.[11] Going vegan is actually quite similar to the Mediterranean diet—it just takes the further step of leaving out meat, eggs, dairy, and other animal-based products, while still providing plenty of glucose for energy and willpower. With a vegan diet, protein comes from legumes like lentils and beans, nuts, and seeds. Fatty acids can come from ground flax seeds (tastier than they sound!) and walnuts. A vitamin B_{12} supplement is highly recommended.

You might try a vegan diet for a week, or at least a few days, and see what you think. You can always go back to corn dogs. (I just hope you won't.)

"WHOSE FORK IS IT, ANYWAY?"

Let's take back control of how much we eat. After all, we have human agency and we're the ones who put fork to mouth. The trouble is that our diet is so deeply influenced by so many external agents—secret agents, to most of us. A big one is the food industry, which has become increasingly adept at leading us around by our dopamine-driven noses, ears, and eyes.

Take names, for example. Sales of chocolate cake, for instance, increase by 27 percent when it's called a "Belgian Black Forest Chocolate Cake" rather than a simple "Chocolate Cake"—never mind that the Black Forest is in Germany, not Belgium.[12] A "Big Gulp" suggests not only a beverage the size of an oil tanker, but the way you should drink it.

But this is America, right? Nobody tells the proud, the many, the fat, how much (or little) to eat. If faced with a gargantuan piece of Belgian Black Forest Chocolate Cake, we eat it and face the consequences later. (The tendency is especially common at cruise ship buffets, where each passenger is offered a plate the size of a small toboggan and encouraged to fill and repeat.) Bigger bowls, plates, and serving spoons all result in taking larger portions, which of course we feel we must finish.[13] And we actually don't mind too much. Our brains don't tell us that we're full until many minutes afterward, so we continue to eat until the last large spoonful of the fist-sized scoop of ice cream is gone. Eat in haste; repent at leisure.

The size of the container can even be more important than the taste of the food. Cornell researcher Brian Wansink and his colleague Kim Junyong discovered that people ate 45 percent more when served fresh popcorn from extra-large containers than from large containers. More amazingly, even when the popcorn was stale (five days old!), they still ate 34 percent more from the extra-large megabuckets. As Wansink observes in his book *Mindless Eating,*[14] "we eat with our eyes."

So now that we're making the secret agents controlling our diet not so secret, let's exert our own agency and take control of how much we eat by serving ourselves portion sizes that are reasonable.

Do we really want to let all that food on our plate go to waste? No. We could wrap it up for a future meal or snack. If a dessert simply looks too good to pass up, well, don't pass it up, but take only a few bites and bring the rest home for a dessert the next night.

Or give it to a homeless person on the street:

"Spare some change for food?"

"Well, actually, I don't have any change, but I do have half a piece of Belgian Black Forest Chocolate Cake. It looks really good and it's still the size of a schnauzer."

"Thanks, man!"

No joke. I love to try the taste of a dessert but not necessarily get stuffed to the gills on it.

Now it's time to upset my mom . . .

DOWN WITH THE CLEAN-PLATE CLUB!

We could get control over the portions of food we eat—but it isn't something we learned as children. Most of us of a certain age remember the "clean-plate club," or the guilt-inducing aphorism, "Clean your plate because there are starving children around the world." Did our mothers want us to become obese and have no energy? Because that's what we did.

Now let's upset nutritionists, too . . .

UP WITH SNACKING!

Many nutritionists still tell us to avoid snacking. They are, for the most part, wrong. To keep glucose levels more or less constant throughout the day (and not become like the hypoglycemic judges mentioned earlier), you might consider noshing on fruit, vegetables, yogurt, low-fat cottage cheese, nuts, sunflower or pumpkin seeds, or trail mix.

A recent study following over four hundred New Zealand college students for thirteen days found that both fruit and vegetable intake was associated with more purpose in life and creativity.[15] One reason for this, the researchers suggest, may be that B vitamins from fruits and vegetables increase the functioning of mitochondria—the power plants of our cells—stimulating greater energy and engagement.[16]

At JOOL Health we make snacks like these freely available through the day. Snacks, combined with standing desks, a meditation and nap room, and a yoga room, have resulted in an extremely productive work environment.

EAT FOR LIFE

Finally, let's not forget what we're *not* here for: to become skinny models or hypervigilant health nuts who worry about everything they consume. People who talk about their LDL cholesterol numbers or the calories they consume are, at least to me, boring. With apologies to John Lennon:

> But if you go counting the calories in your chow,
> You ain't gonna make it with anyone, anyhow!

There's no need to be excessive about diet—in either direction. Fittingly, Aristotle proposed a golden mean for diet: "If we drink or eat too much, that will destroy our health, whereas drinking and eating proportionate amounts creates, increases, and preserves it."[17] Many of the most purposeful people I know find a way to maintain a reasonable, enjoyable, well-balanced diet. Because they have big purposes, they're busy people . . . which means that they may cook a bit themselves but often don't have time to shop, prepare, cook, and clean up, so they take out food or go out to eat.

If that describes you, the Mediterranean diet may still be a good fit. If you're taking out or eating out, consider choosing places that specialize in various Middle Eastern cuisines.

SIMPLE TIPS FOR EATING WELL

There are thousands of good eating tips. The ones that follow are designed to give you more energy and willpower for . . . what? That's right, for daily living toward an awesome purpose.

- Eat slowly. Pause now and then to check in on your satisfaction level. Smell the food. Then taste it. If you catch yourself taking the express train rather than the local, try putting your fork down after each bite.
- Approaching each meal armed with a scale and a calorie chart is a good way to improve your diet—and lose

your friends. With the Mediterranean diet in mind, fill half your plate with vegetables, a fourth with a protein (fish, lean meat, beans, lentils, etc.), and the rest with a healthy starch (potato, rice, pasta, etc.).

- Eat light and eat often. This will maintain blood glucose for energy and willpower without causing dramatic peaks and valleys.

- If you have a choice (for example, in your own house), control portion sizes by using smaller plates and glasses. Remember what Brian Wansink says: "We eat with our eyes."

- Try to avoid multitasking at the table; the distractions make it easy to go on autopilot. As anyone knows who's gotten up from a full season of *Game of Thrones* and found himself knee-deep in empty pizza boxes, binge watching is often accompanied by binge eating.

- Try lemon on cantaloupe, balsamic vinegar and fresh basil on tomato slices, or if you're feeling ambitious, a lime-based vegetarian seviche. And for a real taste sensation, drizzle warm balsamic vinegar on raspberry sorbet. No, really.

- "Drive off the top of the tank." Instead of waiting till you're running on fumes, then screeching into a gas station to fill 'er up, make each meal just big enough to get you through the next few hours. There's even an added bonus: your next meal will come that much sooner!

- While everyone else is arguing over whether it's called

"soda" or "pop," reach for a cool, clear glass of water and sit back as they duke it out. To jazz things up, add a little fruit juice for color and flavor.

- Ditch those unhealthy carbs and load up on beans instead. Turns out beans are packed with protein and fiber, making them good for your heart and digestive tract.

- Fiber is your friend. Keep things moving through your digestive pipeline with a generous daily intake of whole grains, fruits, vegetables, beans, peas, and nuts.

- "Dinner is not a feast, it is a ceremony," said Irish wit Oscar Wilde.[18] We're not sure we'd go that far, but there can be a lot more to a meal than snarfing Hot Pockets while scanning Instagram. Set the scene, dim the lights, savor each bite. With all that going on, you might eat less and enjoy it more.

- With a little effort you can train your sweet tooth to desert dessert. It's expecting some sugar as a signal that you're done eating. Don't overindulge it! A piece of ripe fruit or a square of dark chocolate (eaten as slowly as humanly possible) just might do the trick.

- Sugar can be sneaky! Look for it hiding in your food under other names on the ingredients list of packaged foods—ingredients like high fructose corn syrup, cane syrup, or any of several other nasty characters with names ending in -ose.

- Cutting out refined sugar is a good thing, but not all

at once—going "cold turkey" can result in low energy, shaking, and headaches. Instead, cut back in phases: get used to each reduction before moving on to the next.

- Don't skimp on the cinnamon! It's a tasty natural "sweetener" and has been shown to regulate blood sugar and help control appetite. Add it to your yogurt, coffee, or entrees (especially Indian food).

- Acquiring a taste for the unfamiliar (like feta or kale) may take time, but it's worth the effort. And getting used to smaller portions of something *familiar* (like sugar) works the same way. It can take ten to twenty tries to develop a new taste preference. We're not talking love at first bite here, but over time you can truly begin to enjoy a healthier diet.

- Sometimes the simplest solutions are the best. Drinking a glass of water before each meal (1) makes you feel fuller, so you eat less; (2) keeps you hydrated; and (3) works wonders for your skin.

- It's no secret that more and more restaurants are "supersizing" their portions . . . or that eating those portions will likely supersize *you*. Fight upselling by asking for a to-go box as you order. Not only does this help reduce portion size, but it provides another great meal for later.

- One benefit of the celebrity-chef and online-recipe explosion is the sudden availability of healthier versions of old favorites. Try swapping in cauliflower for potatoes, non-

fat yogurt for sour cream, unsweetened applesauce for
sugar—the substitutions and flavor sensations are endless.

- Craving a carbonated soft drink? Reach for seltzer water
  instead. Even diet soda is loaded with stuff you don't
  want in your body. Seltzer comes in lots of flavors without added sugar or chemicals, and it's just as bubbly.

- Going vegetarian at least one meal a week sparks culi-
  nary creativity and saves money. Think globally—most
  other countries eat less meat than Americans, and the
  way international recipes use grains, nuts, and vegetables will blow your mind instead of your budget.

- Pack your lunch and unpack some pounds. Bringing
  your lunch to work likely means a healthier and more
  balanced meal than what you'd get at a restaurant.

- Not all fats are created equal. Saturated fats—like the
  ones that come from meat and dairy products—stay
  solid at room temperature. Unsaturated fats—from
  nuts, seeds, grains, fish, and some vegetables—don't.
  Focus more on foods that contain unsaturated fats
  when possible and see if you experience a difference in
  how you feel.

- At the grocery store, decrease your diameter by shopping the perimeter. Fresh foods are often found out at
  the edges, while processed foods full of fat and sugar
  line the aisles. Outsmart the marketing wizards by
  avoiding the middle; your middle will thank you.

- When possible, eat locally sourced, seasonal produce. It supports the economy where you live and nourishes you with a variety of fresh, field-to-table nutrients.

This chapter focused on eating in a way that helps you build a sustainable diet for daily energy and willpower. But my recommendations could turn some people off. Eating in this way is difficult if you live in a "food desert" (an urban area where it's hard to find fresh, healthy food), if you can't afford certain foods, or if you don't have time or know how to cook.

Yet many economically poor people I meet in other countries actually do eat like this: less meat and more fresh fruits and vegetables. In fact, when such people move to the United States, they tend to quickly become overweight. Poor people in America used to starve. Now, with the availability of cheap, convenient, unhealthful fast food, they don't starve, but they get sick and die far before their time from diabetes, heart disease, and other diet-related illnesses.

Teaching basic cooking skills and making healthier foods available are important public health efforts. A related effort is to help individuals become more resilient in these difficult environments. And as we'll see in the next chapter, resiliency—like so many other things— flows from purpose.

Four

LEARNING TO SAIL

13

SAILING THROUGH STORMS

"Learning how to think" really means learning how
to exercise control over *how* and *what* you think.
It means being conscious and aware enough to
choose what you pay attention to and to choose
how to construct meaning from experience.
Because if you cannot or will not exercise this kind
of choice in adult life, you will be totally hosed.

—DAVID FOSTER WALLACE[1]

PEOPLE SHAKING UP THE WORLD

As I've mentioned before, my field of public health takes me all over the world. But in all my travels, I've never worked with individuals so poor in material goods yet so rich in *life* as the people of Africa.

A number of people I've worked with there are now dead from AIDS or malaria or tuberculosis. An AIDS worker I'd met and befriended was tragically killed a few months later by an undetected land mine. And yet Africa is where I've met the kindest people I've ever known.

I've met people who laugh, make incredible music, and party like Keith Richards. A man I'd just met cooked and shared with me the only chicken he and his family will eat for months. I've danced and played conga drums late into the night with a band in the remote Zambian bushland until a fellow musician whispered to me gently, "You know man, you play just like a Swede!" I grinned and gave him an alcohol-lubed "Thanks!"—only to realize later that it wasn't a compliment. It was just the nicest way he could say that I had absolutely no rhythm.*

When people tell me that finding purpose is a first-world problem—a higher-order concern, only to be dealt with once other important needs such as safety, food, shelter, education, and self-esteem have been met—I immediately think of the people of Africa, many of whom grew up with none of these benefits. Yet they still have a purpose.

The scientist: When Esther Ngumbi discovered the world of science as a child, she knew that she wanted to live in that world. Raised in a rural community in Kenya, Esther defied the status quo and earned her PhD in entomology (insect research). "As I walked up to the podium to receive my doctoral degree," she told me, "my thoughts meandered back to Kenya. I thought of the many children in my community who had the potential to be a scientist like me but lacked the opportunity. It was during that day that I told myself, I would do whatever it would take to give the children in my community, the children from other poor communities, the children in Africa the opportunities so that they can break the poverty barrier, get an education and go out to attain whatever it is that they want to become."

After becoming a researcher at Auburn University in the United States, Esther decided to return to her Kenyan community and start a library. She began by collecting books from Auburn. "I was deter-

---

* My sincerest apologies to all of the great Swedish drummers! Particularly Tomas Haake, drummer for the metal band *Meshuggah,* and Morgan Ågren, who drummed for *Fläskkvartetten* (Fleshquartet) and sat in on Dweezil Zappa's sweet album *Shampoohorn.*

mined to carry these books to Kenya, come rain or come sunshine."[2] Loaded down like a Sherpa, she arrived at the ticket desk of the Atlanta airport, only to be told that she was forty pounds over her allowance for checked luggage.

> So I quickly packed the books in my *hand* luggage. Then in Dubai, I was changing to a Kenya Airlines flight. Five minutes before flight, a person came up to me and said, "Excuse me, young lady, did you know that every passenger on Kenya Airlines can carry only five pounds?" So I literally walked up to every passenger and said, "EXCUSE ME, I'm a student. I believe in inspiring our younger generation. If you believe in education, if you believe in inspiring the next generation, please, have a book, help me take these books to Kenya!"
> Some people took my books. Others just stared at me blankly. *"Crazy Kenyan lady!"*

She was able to get fellow passengers to take thirty-five pounds of the books but still had five remaining extra pounds.

> So as I was boarding the plane, the guy taking tickets said, "I'm sorry, but you still have ten pounds. You can only take five pounds." I looked at him back and I said, *"EXCUSE ME, if you believe in inspiring young Kenyans, don't argue with me, just let me on the plane!"*

He let her on the plane.

"For the love of young Kenyans," Esther said, "I am determined to do anything and everything until it comes to a better end. I may have looked crazy and stupid in Dubai, but in this business of development, you have to be undaunted."

Esther told me that she now wants to give courage to others. "I have come to realize that many of them are hidden leaders—meaning that they are individuals whose leadership capacity is limited by the suppression of their ideas, insights, knowledge and skills. As we equip them with the knowledge and skills, as well as creating an environment necessary for them to thrive, we see them starting to realize their purpose. They begin to appreciate their talents, gifts and abilities. Afterwards, the rest becomes history."

The educator: By the time James Arinaitwe was ten, he was labeled an "AIDS orphan." "My grandmother, who raised me after my parents both died, literally devoted her life to leaving a legacy in the world. She's an obstetrician with no formal education. She'd wake up in the middle of the night to help women give birth. I once asked her, 'Why do you do this?' 'Obuntu [humanity],' she replied. 'I believe that each child I deliver could save another person's life.' This is the lesson she taught me."

James traveled over three hundred miles—on foot—from western Uganda to the president of Uganda's residential home "because my grandma and I had heard that he was helping orphans like myself attend school . . . I was met by the first lady of the country who graciously offered a scholarship to a private school in Kampala for my high school education." He now has a master's degree in public health and is the cofounder and executive director of Teach for Uganda, a not-for-profit organization working to ensure that "one day all Ugandan children, despite their socio-economic status or family background, will receive an excellent and equitable education."

"I have two purposes," James told me. "The first one is to leave behind a world where everyone who's been denied opportunity can achieve their dreams and vision in life." The second? "Whenever I meet someone, I want to leave them to think, 'This person made me feel better today! I feel like I met a wonderful human being.'"

Clearly none of these accomplishments came easily. His exposure to the modern American diet didn't help, either. "In the United States while getting my master's degree, I started eating more processed foods, frozen foods, and fast food. I could also get all of these refills of soft drinks. No wonder my whole body crashed! I changed my diet to include more vegetables and fruit—the kind of food I used to eat in Uganda. It changed my life! No more problems."

James laughed when I asked him whether purpose in life was really relevant to those who had so many other needs. "Families that break down are the ones who have no purpose or vision for the family. Purpose goes hand in hand with hope. Hope for their children. Hope for a better life. In the West, people may not relate to this, but this is how we think. Purpose sustains poor people."

The advocate: "Without a purpose in my life, I would have committed suicide a long time ago," Henry Nyombi told me. At the age of twelve, he was hit by an overloaded pickup truck as he was walking to school in Uganda. He was left a permanent wheelchair user in a country not recognized for its support of people with disabilities.

After losing his father to cancer when Henry was nine and his mother from yellow fever when he was twelve, Henry faced his new-found disability as an orphan. He went through his country's educational system facing a physically inaccessible environment and no legal framework to protect him, coupled with harsh treatment from teachers and fellow students.

"Uganda has a stigma against those with disabilities, and I realized that I would need to help myself," he told me, "so I decided to set goals that I wanted to achieve over time. Every day, I would take a step back and reflect on my goals. The trauma of my disability affected my sleep, but my goals would console me and encourage me and allowed me to sleep better."

Today Henry is a lawyer and serves as chairperson for the National Union of Disabled Persons of Uganda. He's also director of the Youth with Physical Disability Development Forum, a community-based organization that enables youth with physical disabilities to enjoy equal rights in society and realize full social and educational inclusion.

"My purpose is to see that Uganda has a legal framework that protects marginalized people, including women and children and youth and people with disabilities. To see the world become an open society that appreciates everyone."

Talking with Henry, I felt that anything that doesn't kill him just makes him stronger. He told me, "When many people I know think about their history, they get nightmares and ask themselves 'Why me, why me, why me?' I don't waste my time thinking about problems. One could reflect on their history and break down. I didn't do that. I motivate myself because I have a goal to achieve. I turn my history into lessons."

PEOPLE SHAKEN UP BY THE WORLD

There are now literally thousands of studies examining resilience to traumatic events and difficult circumstances, with many connections to purpose in life, energy, willpower, and SPACE behaviors. I'll illustrate relevant findings through the studies of three earthquakes.

Why earthquakes? Because movement and devastation from the very ground we walk on, I believe, shakes us to our existential bones. There are few things we rely on more than the stability of *terra firma,* and people respond very differently when they "quake in their boots." For this reason, earthquake epicenters have been a favorite destination for resilience researchers.

Earthquake one: On October 8, 2005, at 8:50 A.M., the most devastating temblor to strike Pakistan in the last century killed over 250,000 people and left more than 3.5 million homeless.

In its aftermath, a team of researchers from multiple U.S. universities[3] interviewed 200 survivors, the majority of whom had lost at least one relative and over 80 percent of whom had become homeless. They found that roughly 65 percent were suffering from posttraumatic stress disorder (PTSD). But 35 percent were not.

What separated the two groups? Was it whether a loved one had died in the earthquake? The proximity to the epicenter? Partially, but stronger than either factor was whether the person had a strong sense of purpose in life. Purpose in life was associated with both lower PTSD and depressive symptoms.

Earthquake two: On May 12, 2008, at 2:28 P.M., a powerful earthquake shook the Sichuan Province of China, causing approximately 70,000 deaths and over 370,000 injuries and leaving as many as 11 million people homeless.

One year later, researchers and their survey teams interviewed over 2,000 survivors.[4] The researchers were monitoring PTSD from the quake's effects, but they were also looking for the opposite: post-traumatic *growth*. Did the experience improve the survivors' relations with others? Did it improve their psychological strength? Did they begin considering new possibilities? Did they have a greater appreciation of life?

Refusing to conform to the status quo view of stress, over *half* of the survivors reported significant personal growth from the experience. Further defying conventional wisdom, the researchers found that those experiencing the greatest growth were the *most* affected by the earthquake. Post-traumatic growth protected the survivors from future PTSD, as well.[5]

Five years out, another research team came back to study the long-term outcomes of the survivors. They still found post-traumatic growth and learned that it was related to individuals' expressions of *energy* and *willpower*.[6] Sound familiar?

Earthquake three: On March 11, 2011, at 2:46 P.M., the fourth-most-powerful earthquake in recorded history hit the Tohoku region of Japan, resulting in over 15,000 deaths and over 6,000 injuries and leaving almost a quarter of a million people homeless. A tsunami caused by the earthquake triggered meltdowns in three reactors of the Fukushima Daiichi Nuclear Power Plant, requiring the evacuation of hundreds of thousands more residents. The release of radioactive material, the largest since the 1986 Chernobyl meltdown, created tremendous anxiety throughout the region.

Three months after the event, researchers surveyed over 1,000 survivors who were near the epicenter. They found that, even more than the disaster itself, people's *interpretations* of the disaster had a strong influence on their outcomes.[7] Those who viewed the traumatic event as something that frightened them or damaged their lives were likely to suffer from stress, depression, and a lower quality of life. On the other hand, those viewing the event as a *challenge* that they could learn from were more likely to develop post-traumatic growth and a *higher* quality of life.

Two years after the earthquake, a separate group of researchers interviewed over three hundred Japanese students living within two hundred miles of the epicenter.[8] The researchers thought that a disaster such as the Tohoku earthquake would prompt the students to reexamine their core beliefs and assumptions about the world and raise such questions as, "Is there order in the world?" and "Is the world 'good' or 'fair'?" We might assume that people who had their core beliefs dramatically shaken by this horrific incident would suffer more than grow. Yet those who had their beliefs most disrupted experienced the *greatest* post-traumatic growth.

What lessons can we draw from these studies of purpose and resilience?

PURPOSE AND RESILIENCE

First, it's our interpretation of, and approach to, our past that generates resilience. The existential philosopher Jean-Paul Sartre went even further, saying not only that we interpret our past but that this interpretation flows from what he called our "fundamental project"—basically, our purpose in life.

The cases at the beginning of the chapter illustrate this process. Henry Nyombi's purpose—to protect people with disabilities—influences how he views his past. His interpretation of his history then becomes the message sent to the marginalized people he's serving: "Do not become a victim of *your* past!"

Viewing an earthquake's devastation as a challenge to be met squarely, rather than run from, was also found to promote post-traumatic growth and quality of life. In fact, studies of both the Sichuan, China, and Tohoku, Japan, earthquake survivors found that greater challenges promoted *more* growth.

Second, resilience occurs when you stop being afraid and start being yourself. Esther Ngumbi said that she "may have looked crazy and stupid." Crazy and stupid? I see her as courageous . . . and so did many of her fellow passengers. Esther isn't daunted by, or afraid of, the opinions of others—she runs on pure, unadulterated purpose. Fear reduces resilience and the ability to grow from trauma, and purposeful living reduces fear.

Studies have shown that first affirming core values reduces a fearful response to a threat.[9] A neuroimaging study[10] found that individuals with a strong purpose in life have less volatile responses to negative events from their amygdala, the part of our brains associated with fear and anxiety. Purpose in life also predicts smaller eyeblinks from negative images—an indicator of better emotional recovery.[11] It even improves our ability to cope with pain.[12]

Third, traumatic events that shatter one's world can also lead to a reexamination of one's perception of the world. *This can be a good thing.* None of us wants to be shattered, whether from illness, divorce, losing a job, or losing a loved one, but this trauma can let us see things from a fresh perspective, allowing us to "repurpose" our lives.

And finally, purposeful living is for everyone, regardless of socioeconomic status. It's well established that society's poor and disadvantaged suffer more from chronic physical and mental illnesses than do its rich and advantaged. Everyone experiences stress, but being poor means having fewer resources to cope with it. Studies have shown that the effects of poverty and racism can actually reduce one's *ability* to deal with stress.[13] But as the aforementioned stories illustrate, this isn't the case for everyone. What makes the difference?

Northwestern University psychologists Edith Chen and Greg Miller suggest that two factors, when combined, can help a person defend against stress. They call their model "shift-and-persist." By accepting, and adjusting to, the stressors of life—by making a *shift* in perception—we benefit. Sometimes fighting against every stressor in our environment can be like struggling in quicksand: it just sinks you deeper.

But this shift in perception must be accompanied by a *persistent* pursuit of a goal—as James Arinaitwe called it earlier in this chapter, a "hope for a better life." Studies of this shift-and-persist approach have been very promising, demonstrating improved control over obesity[14] and asthma[15] as well as the regulation of inflammation.[16]

One could therefore argue that purpose in life is not only available to the poor but *essential* to their very survival. As James Arinaitwe suggested, purpose "sustains the poor." The most affirmative responses to the World Values Survey question, "Do you think about the meaning and purpose of life?" come from some of the most impoverished countries in the world, including Colombia, Ghana, Indonesia, and Rwanda.[17] The same survey, when conducted in the United States, revealed that those who in the last twelve months had gone without enough to eat, felt unsafe from crime, gone without needed medicines or medical treatments, or who had gone without a cash income thought more about purpose than those who hadn't. Purpose, as James Arinaitwe said, goes hand in hand with hope.

What Viktor Frankl called our "will to meaning" is common among all humans, even those in the direst circumstances. Mohamed Abdulkadir Ali writes of a twenty-two-year-old man named Liban, who made the exceedingly dangerous trip from Somalia to Europe: "Like many of [his fellow migrants], Liban did not face persecution or danger, just a life without purpose or hope. That is why he and thousands of others have risked their lives each year, and will continue to do so despite the recent headlines about hundreds of migrants drowned."[18]

BROKEN OPEN

"The only reason I keep my head above water is because I have a goal in life that I am determined to reach," wrote my daughter Julia to a student from her high school. This theme runs through many studies of patients with cancer,[19] heart disease, stroke,[20] diabetes, spinal cord injury,[21] tuberculosis,[22] and multiple sclerosis,[23] among other illnesses. Purpose in life provides resilience to people going through long- and short-term illnesses.

The positive "breaking open" effect found in the people reexamining their core beliefs after the Tohoku earthquake and tsunami has also been found among leukemia patients going through chemotherapy.[24] When Ram Dass, Harvard psychologist-turned–spiritual– teacher, suffered a severe stroke at sixty-five, he regarded the stroke as an "act of grace," saying, *"Ego breaks open—then you see who you really are!"*[25]

Having a purpose doesn't guarantee a one-hundred-year life span. Sometimes it's nineteen years. But however long our life is, or whatever we go through, we can look at purposeful living as a way to give us greater resilience, and possibly even growth.

Now it's time to connect the dots . . .

14

AN EXCELLENT SAILOR

The life we receive is not short, but we make it so,
nor do we have any lack of it, but are wasteful of it.

SENECA[1]

One of the reasons I went to meet with a Vedanta Hindu guru in northern India was to ask a question.

After Julia died, I started seeing her eye—her actual eye—in my meditation sessions. With my own eyes shut, as I went into a deeper meditative state, my inner vision would see her wide-open eye—alive, looking peacefully at me. It seemed like my meditation was creating a portal to . . . somewhere?

"Do you think it's her? Is it my daughter?" I asked the guru, trying to rein in my emotions. The white-suited man smiled gently and said, "Well, yes and no. She's now in a very different place. At the same time, she's in you, in your heart. Always. This is what you are seeing."

Where this "very different place" was, I didn't bother asking: Was she an octopus in the ocean? Someone's kitchen flatware? Was she occupying nine dimensions of space? But the guru was right—Julia still lives in me.

This is difficult to explain using the methods of science.

Stephen Hawking said that "philosophy is dead" and that "scientists have become the bearers of the torch of discovery in our quest for knowledge."[2] But what is philosophy, anyway? Isaac Newton and other scientists of the seventeenth-century Royal Society were called "philosophers." The term simply means "lover of wisdom." It doesn't mean astrologer, palm reader, or witch burner. It's someone who's unafraid to ask the big questions.

As a scientist I know that our tools provide an effective way of answering many questions, but I wonder whether we're the *only* "bearers of the torch of discovery" that Hawking speaks of. Friedrich Nietzsche said, "A 'scientific' interpretation of the world, as you understand it, might . . . be one of the *most stupid* of all possible interpretations of the world, meaning that it would be one of the poorest in meaning."[3] Nietzsche was saying that science reduces nature to a description of its mechanical parts, and when one does this, everything starts looking like a machine . . . including us.

But can we understand, from the sum of its mechanical parts, the comfort given by a nurse holding a patient's hand being wheeled into surgery? Or a sunset? Or a kiss? Or a piece of music? Nietzsche actually uses music as an example: "Assuming that one estimated the *value* of a piece of music according to how much of it could be counted, calculated, and expressed in formulas: how absurd would such a 'scientific' estimation of music be. What would one have comprehended, understood, grasped of it? Nothing, really nothing of what is 'music' in it!"

Whether we're machines or not, scientists can study the concept of purpose in life as they would study music. Unable to reduce it to a set of mechanical parts, they can still examine its effects. With conceptualizations of purpose that have for thousands of years been framed by philosophy (such as eudaimonia), scientists have learned a great deal over the past decade about how to live a happier, healthier life. It's this knowledge that I've attempted to organize in this book.

WHAT WE KNOW

And what's the verdict? I think we have enough evidence to support the following conclusions:

- A strong, transcending purpose in life is good for your health and well-being and protects against disease and death.
- Purpose is a high-level goal (which is motivating) that is deeply valued (which is also motivating).
- The *type* of values that constitute a purpose matters.
- A strong, transcending purpose in life reduces defensiveness to change.
- Your purpose in life might be revealed by God . . . but it might not (hardly a conclusion!).
- Purposeful living is a dynamic process that requires energy and willpower.
- Five positive behaviors that can improve energy and willpower are sleep, presence, activity, creativity, and eating well (SPACE).

- Purposeful living is not just a higher-order aspiration for the well-heeled. It's for everyone.

WHAT WE DON'T KNOW

We still don't know very much about interventions meant to increase purpose in life, let alone their results. The interventions that have been developed and tested have shown positive results, but they tend to require significant interactions with therapists and are focused on patients with serious illnesses or other problems.

How can we democratize purpose-in-life interventions? Books (such as this one) could be thought of as interventions for the public, but their effect hasn't been studied scientifically. In an attempt to reach a broad spectrum of people, I've been working with colleagues to develop apps for the Web and for smartphones that help people develop purpose and monitor energy, willpower, and SPACE behaviors. Ultimately the scientific community will determine the impact of these and other similar interventions.

BUT FOR NOW . . .

If I were you, I wouldn't wait around for more research. I'd just get a purpose. The scientific evidence supporting the benefits of one is extremely promising, and at the risk of sounding a bit alarmist, *we need it*.

You may be thinking at this point, "That's easy for you to say, buddy; you've already got a purpose that works for you. What about the rest of us?" Touché. I had to go through a lot (much of which I would have been happy to skip) to find a personal, meaningful purpose that guides and inspires me every day. But you can find one, too. And at the risk of sounding a bit cavalier, the specific nature of your purpose is less important than the *fact that you have one.*

Afraid you might pick a clunker the first time out? Maybe you will. But remember, you've got your friends, your family, your intelligence, your culture, your values, and above all your conscience to guide you. It's unlikely you'll miss the mark by much.

And if you do . . . so what? Remember, unlike your past (or for that matter, most tattoos), your purpose *can be easily changed*! You can refine, update, edit, expand, reduce, or overhaul it any time you like. In fact, I've done all of these things over the years, and my purpose—and life—is a lot better for it.

The opposite of a self-transcending purpose is narcissism (excessive interest in oneself) and nihilism (the belief that life has no purpose). I'm concerned about the surge of both in our society. A 1966 survey of American college freshmen found that 42 percent thought it was very important to be well-off financially and 86 percent thought it was very important to have a meaningful philosophy of life. But in 2005 these statistics essentially reversed, with 75 percent now believing that it's very important to be well-off financially and only 46 percent believing it very important to have a meaningful philosophy of life.[4] This shift from the existential to the material is, I believe, a major source of discontent in our society.

In my own experience as a teacher, I've never seen students who were so focused on success but at the same time so anxious, depressed, and lonely as they seem now. Economic growth in the United States has not made us happier.[5] And when we get off the hamster wheel for a brief moment, we don't even know what to do with our lives. As Bertrand Russell lamented, "What will be the good of the conquest of leisure and health, if no one remembers how to use them?"[6]

But many of us *are* trying to remember what to do with our lives. Since 2008, adjusting for sheer volume, Google searches for the phrase *purpose in life* have more than doubled, as have the number of research studies related to it. As I travel around the world speaking, I'm heartened by the interest in the subject. After every presentation individuals approach me with questions about getting their son, their mother, their friend, or themselves connected with a purpose bigger than themselves.

Through these presentations I've also been privileged to meet hundreds of people who have lost loved ones. I can usually see it in their faces as they approach me after a talk—they're in "the club." Just as a woman wrote to the Stoic philosopher Seneca two thousand years ago asking what she should do with her raging, continuing grief over the loss of her sixteen-year-old son,[7] members of the club know that the sadness doesn't go away.

There are times during the day that I still cry and physically ache over the loss of Julia. Many nights I have dreams in which she's a young girl, playing. I feel an overwhelming urge to protect her, then suddenly wake up realizing that she doesn't need my protection anymore.

Yet in a strange way, I know that this grief has led me to becoming a happier person. I also see it in other parents who've lost children. Of course, they're not happier in the hedonic, "I have a new toy" sense; they're happier in the eudaimonic, "I have a new life" sense. They've been broken open and they now see more clearly.[8]

Like my third-century hero, Saint Lawrence, who was slowly grilled alive for giving the church's riches to the poor, I'd like to think that I can face, and even tease, what is tormenting me: *"I'm well done. Turn me over!"* Regardless of what's happened, I get to choose who I am. Just as Aimee Mullins refused to change the dress that exposed her wooden legs, she will "decide, and decide again" who she's going to be . . . just as Henry Nyombi gets to turn his history of struggle and discrimination into "lessons."

We are who we choose to be, so we should be *very careful* who we choose to be. During the course of our lives, we're likely to struggle with decisions over a career, fret over a boring job, hope to reengage with our partner, wonder what to do when our teenager stays out until 3:00 A.M., attempt to enjoy Thanksgiving when sitting next to our jerk of a brother-in-law, and try to figure out how to live to—and live through—a ripe old age.

A purpose, driven by self-transcending core values, isn't a panacea. But it *can* provide guidance with the choices we make throughout our lives, whether it's one's career, engaging in a job, reaffirming a wedding vow, understanding a teenager, finding shared values leading to an interesting conversation over turkey and mashed potatoes, and tolerating—perhaps even enjoying—old age as opposed to becoming

George Bernard Shaw's "feverish selfish little clod of ailments and grievances."[9]

THE LAKE

In the summer evening I settle into my kayak and paddle out onto Lake Michigan. Watching the sun melt into the calm water, I still feel Julia in me. She's in my loving-kindness meditation. We look at the sunset together and smile, and I wish her peace and happiness.

Lately, the family portion of my purpose ("to be an engaged husband and father") has required an important revision: I've added *"and grandfather,"* with the birth of Madeleine Julia, my daughter Rachael's new baby. That's one of the nice things about life: like family, like compassion, like understanding, like a rubber band, it can be wonderfully elastic.

The line in Lucretius's poem *On the Nature of Things* is as relevant now as it was over two thousand years ago:

> While some are ascendant, some recede, and generations are renewed again in a brief space, passing life's torch, like relay runners in a race.

Thanks to a numerical coincidence, my teaching career blesses me with a poignant gift: every year I'm blessed with a new crop of students who are just the age that Julia reached at the end of her brief, big life. I enjoy watching each succeeding generation ascend, with a commitment to finding purpose in their lives.

Five years before, at this very place on Lake Michigan, I wasn't thinking and wasn't caring about myself or anyone else. Then, I felt Julia telling me that if I was to survive, I would need to *get over myself* and *live for what matters most*.

I've found a breeze at my back and a gentle current. And I know what harbor to make for. I have a lot to do before I die.

Acknowledgments

THE ADVICE AND ENCOURAGEMENT OF MY FRIEND MONTE Montgomery was essential in seeing this book to fruition. My wife, Jeri, gave me the solitary time and support required for research and writing. My daughter Rachael, through her work at the New Voices Fellowship program of the Aspen Institute, provided an avenue to interact with the three individuals whose stories were told in chapter 13. Gideon Weil, my editor at HarperOne, provided continual guidance and wisdom.

Many of the ideas I present were stimulated by my interactions with Jim Loehr at the Human Performance Institute. His early insights have now been supported by over a decade of research. Moreover, this book couldn't have been written without the efforts of the researchers who study this complex, important, and fascinating area. Special thanks go to my research colleagues Emily Falk and Yoona Kang at the University of Pennsylvania,

Eric Kim at Harvard University, and Ken Resnicow at the University of Michigan.

Sean Foy at the Personal Wellness Corporation provided valuable advice about physical activity for chapter 10. Ari Weinzweig at Zingerman's and Ryan Picarella at WELCOA helped me think through issues of purpose in organizations.

Finally, I'd like to express my deepest gratitude to the hundreds of individuals over the past two years who shared with me their stories of loss, resilience, and purpose.

Notes

CHAPTER 1: CROSSROADS

1. L. Tolstoy, "My Confession," in *The Complete Works of Count Tolstoy,* vol. 13 (Boston: Colonial Press): 18.

2. V. Frankl, *Man's Search for Meaning* (Boston: Beacon Press, 2006): 76.

3. S. Kierkegaard, *The Journals of Kierkegaard 1834–1854,* trans. and ed. Alexander Dru (Fontana: 1958), 44, from Gilleleie, August 1, 1835.

4. P. L. Hill and N. A. Turiano, "Purpose in Life as a Predictor of Mortality Across Adulthood," *Psychological Science* 25, no. 7 (2014): 1482–86.

5. A. H. Mokdad, J. S. Marks, D. F. Stroup, and J. L. Gerberding, "Actual Causes of Death in the United States, 2000," *Journal of the American Medical Association* 291, no. 10 (2004): 1238–45.

6. E. S. Kim, J. K. Sun, N. Park, L. D. Kubzansky, and C. Peterson, "Purpose in Life and Reduced Risk of Myocardial Infarction Among Older U.S. Adults with Coronary Heart Disease: A Two-Year Follow-Up," *Journal of Behavioral Medicine,* February 2012.

7. E. S. Kim, J. K. Sun, N. Park, and C. Peterson, "Purpose in Life and Reduced Incidence of Stroke in Older Adults: The Health and Retirement Study," *Journal of Psychosomatic Research* 74 (2013): 427–32.

8. P. A. Boyle, A. S. Buchman, L. L. Barnes, and D. A. Bennett, "Effect of a Purpose in Life on Risk of Incident Alzheimer Disease and Mild Cognitive Impairment in Community-Dwelling Older Persons," *Archives of General Psychiatry* 67, no. 3 (2010): 304–10.

9. P. A. Boyle, A. S. Buchman, R. S. Wilson, L. Yu, J. A. Schneider, and D. A. Bennett, "Effect of Purpose in Life on the Relation Between Alzheimer Dis-

ease Pathologic Changes on Cognitive Function in Advanced Age," *Archives in General Psychiatry* 69, no. 5 (2012): 499–505.

10. B. A. Prairie, M. F. Scheier, K. A. Matthews, C. C. H. Chang, and R. Hess, "A Higher Sense of Purpose in Life Is Associated with Sexual Enjoyment in Midlife Women," *Menopause* 18, no. 8 (2011): 839–44.

11. E. S. Kim, S. D. Hershner, and V. J. Strecher, "Purpose in Life and Incidence of Sleep Disturbances," *Journal of Behavioral Medicine* 38, no. 3 (2015): 590–97.

12. A. M. Wood and S. Joseph, "The Absence of Positive Psychological (Eudemonic) Well-Being as a Risk Factor for Depression: A Ten-Year Cohort Study," *Journal of Affective Disorders* 122 (2010): 213–17.

13. C. K. Holahan and R. Suzuki, "Motivational Factors in Health Promoting Behavior in Later Aging," *Activities, Adaptation & Aging* 30 (2006): 47–60.

14. N. H. Rasmussen, S. A. Smith, J. A. Maxson, M. E. Bernard, S. S. Cha, D. C. Agerter, and N. D. Shah, "Association of HbA1c with Emotion Regulation, Intolerance of Uncertainty, and Purpose in Life in Type 2 Diabetes Mellitus," *Primary Care Diabetes* 7, no. 3 (2013): 213–21.

15. R. A. Martin, S. MacKinnon, J. Johnson, and D. J. Rohsenow, "Purpose in Life Predicts Treatment Outcome Among Adult Cocaine Abusers in Treatment," *Journal of Substance Abuse Treatment* 40, no. 2 (2011): 183–88.

16. J. E. Bower, M. E. Kemeny, S. E. Taylor, and J. L. Fahey "Finding Positive Meaning and Its Association with Natural Killer Cell Cytotoxicity Among Participants in a Bereavement-Related Disclosure Intervention," *Annals of Behavioral Medicine* 25, no. 2 (2003): 146–55.

17. B. L. Fredrickson, K. M. Grewen, K. A. Coffey, S. B. Algoe, A. M. Firestine, J. M. Arevalo, et al. "A Functional Genomic Perspective on Human Well-Being," *Proceedings of the National Academy of Science U.S.A.* 110 (2013): 13684–89.

18. C. D. Ryff, B. Singer, and G. D. Love, "Positive Health: Connecting Well-Being with Biology," *Philosophical Transactions of the Royal Society of London: Biological Sciences*, 359 (2004): 1383–94.

19. E. S. Kim, V. J. Strecher, and C. D. Ryff, "Purpose in Life and Use of Preventive Health Care Services," *Proceedings of the National Academy of Science* 111, no. 46 (2014): 16331–36.

20. E. S. Epel, E. H. Blackburn, et al., "Accelerated Telomere Shortening in Response to Life Stress," *Proceedings of the National Academy of Science* 101, no. 49 (2004): 17312–15.

21. T. L. Jacobs, E. S. Epel, J. Lin, E. H. Blackburn, et al. "Intensive Meditation Training, Immune Cell Telomerase Activity, and Psychological Mediators," *Psychoneuroendocrinology* 36 (2011): 664–81.

CHAPTER 2: ORIGINS OF PURPOSE

1. A note in one of Darwin's early workbooks, written two years following his return from the voyage on board the HMS *Beagle* and in the midst of writing an account of this voyage, cited in D. M. McMahon, *Happiness: A History* (New York: Grove Press, 2006): 410.

2. S. Hawking and L. Mlodinow, *The Grand Design* (New York: Random House, 2010): 5.

3. Interesting, since as the philosopher Kyle Oskvig writes, "Hawking stands out as a shining example of Aristotelian human excellence." K. Oskvig, "Harder, Faster, Stronger—Better: Aristotle's Ethics and Physical Human Enhancement," *Journal of Evolution & Technology* 23, no. 1 (2013): 19–30.

4. P. Bernstein, *Against the Gods: The Remarkable Story of Risk* (New York: John Wiley & Sons, 1996).

5. K. Vonnegut, *Mother Night* (New York: Fawcett Publications / Gold Medal Books, 1961).

6. D. L. Norton, *Personal Destinies: A Philosophy of Ethical Individualism* (Princeton: Princeton Univ. Press, 1976): 5.

7. Interestingly, *daimon* is also the root of the word *demon*, not surprisingly transformed by Western religions to the negative term, given that these religions viewed humans as inherently sinful as opposed to "divine."

8. Aristotle, *Aristotle: Introductory Readings,* trans. T. Irwin and G. Fine (Indianapolis: Hackett Publishing Company, 1996): 200.

9. Norton, *Personal Destinies,* 3.

10. Fredrickson, et al., "A Functional Genomic Perspective on Human Well-Being," 13684–89.

11. Aristotle, *The Politics of Aristotle,* trans. E. Barker (London: Oxford Univ. Press, 1946): 280.

12. C. P. Niemiec, R. M. Ryan, and E. L. Deci, "The Path Taken: Consequences of Attaining Intrinsic and Extrinsic Aspirations in Post-college Life," *Journal of Research in Personality* 43 (2009): 291–306.

13. E. H. Telzer, A. J. Fuligni, M. D. Lieberman, and A. Galvan, "Neural Sensitivity to Eudaimonic and Hedonic Rewards Differentially Predict Adolescent Depressive Symptoms over Time," *Proceedings of the National Academy of Science,* 2014.

14. John Templeton Foundation, *Does the Universe Have a Purpose?,* (includes an interview with Lawrence Krauss), www.templeton.org/purpose/.

CHAPTER 3: OUR BEST PURPOSE

1. Samuel Barber to his mother, in *Letters of Note,* ed. S. Usher (San Francisco: Chronicle Books, 2014): 231.
2. D. Friend, *The Meaning of Life* (Boston: Little, Brown and Company, 1991).
3. V. J. Strecher, G. H. Seijts, G. J. Kok, G. P. Latham, R. Glasgow, B. DeVellis, R. M. Meertens, and D. W. Bulger, "Goal Setting as a Strategy for Health Behavior Change," *Health Education Quarterly* 22 (1995): 190–200.
4. E. Nordern, "Playboy Interview: Stanley Kubrick," quoted in G. D. Phillips, ed., *Stanley Kubrick: Interviews* (Jackson: Univ. Press of Mississippi, 2001): 47.
5. M. Weber, *The Protestant Ethic and the Spirit of Capitalism* (New York: Penguin Books, 2002).
6. World Values Survey, wave 6, 2010–2014, www.worldvaluessurvey.org.
7. Norton, *Personal Destinies.*
8. E. B. Falk, M. B. O'Donnell, C. N. Cascio, F. Tinney, Y. Kang, M. D. Lieberman, S. E. Taylor, L. An, K. Resnicow, and V. J. Strecher, "Self-Affirmation Alters the Brain's Response to Health Messages and Subsequent Behavior Change," *Proceedings of the National Academy of Science U.S.A.* 112, no. 7 (2015): 1977–82.
9. T. F. Heatherton, "Neuroscience of Self and Self-Regulation," *Annual Review of Psychology* 62 (2011): 363–90.

CHAPTER 4: SELF-TRANSCENDENCE

1. V. Frankl, *The Unheard Cry for Meaning: Psychotherapy and Humanism* (New York: Touchstone Books, 1979): 35.
2. S. Usher, *Lists of Note: An Eclectic Collection Deserving of a Wider Audience* (San Francisco: Chronicle Books, 2015): 36.
3. B. Stulberg, "What's the Point?," *Blue Ridge Outdoors,* July 22, 2015, www.blueridgeoutdoors.com/go-outside/whats-the-point/.
4. A. H. Maslow, "The Farther Reaches of Human Nature," *Journal of Transpersonal Psychology* 1, no. 1 (1969): 1–9.
5. A. H. Maslow, *The Farther Reaches of Human Nature* (New York: Viking Press, 1971): 290.
6. Tim Dahlberg, *Here's to John Wooden and a Life Well Lived* (Los Angeles: The Associated Press, 2010).

7.   Kareem Abdul-Jabbar with Mignon McCarthy, *Kareem* (Random House, New York, 1990): 90–94.

8.   Falsely attributed to Vince Lombardi, this quote is attributed to Henry Russell ("Red") Sanders, former football coach at UCLA. See S. J. Overman, "'Winning Isn't Everything. It's the Only Thing': The Origin, Attributions and Influence of a Famous Football Quote," *Football Studies* 2 no. 2 (1999): 77–99.

9.   Richard Benson, *Sporting Wit: Athletic Wisecracks and Champion Comebacks* (West Sussex: Summersdale Publishers, 2005): 142.

10.   D. S. Yeager, M. D. Henderson, D. Paunesku, G. M. Walton, S. D'Mello, B. J. Spitzer, and A. L. Duckworth, "Boring but Important: A Self-Transcendent Purpose for Learning Fosters Academic Self-Regulation," *Journal of Personality and Social Psychology* 107, no. 4 (2014): 559–80.

11.   F. de Waal, "Putting the Altruism Back into Altruism: The Evolution of Empathy," *Annual Review of Psychology* no. 59 (2008): 279–300.

12.   I. B. A. Bartal, J. Decenty, and P. Mason, "Empathy and Pro-social Behavior in Rats," *Science* no. 334 (2011): 1427.

13.   F. Warneken and M. Tomasello "The Roots of Human Altruism," *British Journal of Psychology* 100 (2009): 455–71.

14.   A. Grant, *Give and Take* (New York: Penguin Books, 2013).

15.   A. Weinzweig, *A Lapsed Anarchist's Approach to Building a Great Business* (Ann Arbor, MI: Zingerman's Press, 2010).

16.   R. Sisodia, D. B. Wolfe, and J. Sheth, *Firms of Endearment* (Upper Saddle River, NJ: Prentice Hall, 2014).

17.   J. Collins, *Good to Great* (New York: Harper Business, 2001).

18.   S. Terkel, *Working* (New York: New Press, 1972).

19.   Gallup, *The State of the American Workplace: Employee Engagement Insights for U.S. Business Leaders,* 2013.

20.   A. M. Grant and D. A. Hofmann, "It's Not all About Me: Motivating Hand Hygiene Among Health Care Professionals by Focusing on Patients," *Psychological Science* 22, no. 12 (2011): 1494–99.

21.   J. E. Dutton, G. Debebe, and A. Wrzesniewski, "Being Valued and Devalued at Work: A Social Valuing Perspective," in *Qualitative Organizational Research: Best Papers from the Davis Conference on Qualitative Research,* vol. 3 (Information Age Publishing: 2015).

22.   G. B. Shaw, *Man and Superman: A Comedy and Philosophy,* Epistle Dedicatory (London: Penguin Books, 2001): 7.

23.   B. L. Arnold and L. S. Lloyd, "Harnessing Complex Emergent Metaphors for Effective Communication in Palliative Care: A Multimodal Perceptual Analy-

sis of Hospice Patients' Reports of Transcendence Experiences," *American Journal of Hospice & Palliative Medicine* no. 31 (2014): 292–99.

CHAPTER 5: MIRACLES, GOD, AND THE AFTERLIFE

1. Kierkegaard, *The Journals of Kierkegaard, 1834–1854,* 44.
2. Primarily composed by Tarantino. Q. Tarantino, *Pulp Fiction*, Miramax Films, 1994.
3. M. Conard, "Symbolism, Meaning & Nihilism in Quentin Tarantino's *Pulp Fiction*," *Philosophy Now,* 1997.
4. R. Warren, *The Purpose Driven Life* (Grand Rapids, MI: Zondervan, 2002): 17.
5. F. Nietzsche, *The Gay Science* (New York: Vintage Books, 1974): 228.
6. This tendency has been discussed for centuries in the field of economics, where it's understood that one's value of a single dollar is smaller if you have 1,003 dollars than if you have 5 dollars, and is a core critique of materialistic values.
7. Andrés Roberto Albertsen, "The Relation Between Faith and Ethics in Kierkegaard's *Fear and Trembling,*" *Teología y Cultura* 15, no. 10 (2013): 19–38.
8. David Brooks, "The Road to Depth: Thinking About What Character Is" (lecture, Aspen Ideas Festival, Aspen, CO, 2014).
9. David Brooks and William Deresiewicz, "What Is College For?" (lecture, Aspen Ideas Festival, Aspen, CO, 2015).
10. D. Barker, *The Good Atheist: Living a Purpose-Filled Life Without God* (Berkeley, CA: Ulysses Press, 2011).
11. A. Camus, *Resistance, Rebellion, and Death,* trans. Justin O'Brien, First Vintage Books edition (New York: Random House, 1974): 10.
12. A. Camus, *The Myth of Sisyphus and Other Essays* (New York: Vintage International, 1991): 3.
13. Camus, *The Myth of Sisyphus and Other Essays,* 123.
14. T. May, *Death* (New York: Routledge, 2009).
15. J. L. Borges, *The Aleph and Other Stories* (New York: Penguin Classics, 2000).
16. E. Kübler-Ross, *On Death and Dying: What the Dying Have to Teach Doctors, Nurses, Clergy & Their Own Families* (New York: Scribner, 1969): 13.
17. P. Coelho, "Your Personal Legend: 28th of May 2009," *Paulo Coelho Writer Official Site,* http://paulocoelhoblog.com/2009/05/28/your-personal-legend-28th-of-may-2009/.

CHAPTER 6: ENERGY

1. Aristotle, *Nicomachean Ethics*, trans. Terence Irwin, 2nd ed. (Cambridge: Hackett Publishing Company, Inc. 1999): 9.

2. An organization he cofounded with Jack Groppel.

3. Lucius Annaeus Seneca, *Letters From a Stoic: Letter LXXI – On the Supreme Good*, trans. Richard Mott Gummere, Loeb Classical Library (Cambridge, Mass.: Harvard Univ. Press, 1917): 163.

4. J. E. Loehr and T. Schwartz, *The Power of Full Engagement* (New York: Free Press, 2003).

5. T. M. Thrash, A. J. Elliot, L. A. Maruskin, and S. E. Cassidy, "Inspiration and the Promotion of Well-Being: Tests of Causality and Mediation," *Journal of Personality and Social Psychology* 98, no. 3 (2010): 488–506.

6. N. Takayama, K. Korpela, J. Lee, T. Morikawa, et al., "Emotional, Restorative and Vitalizing Effects of Forest and Urban Environments at Four Sites in Japan," *International Journal of Environmental Research in Public Health* 11 (2014): 7207–30.

7. J. L. Dude, G. C. Williams, N. Ntoumanis, A. Daley, et al., "Effects of a Standard Provision Versus an Autonomy Supportive Exercise Referral Programme on Physical Activity, Quality of Life and Well-Being Indicators: A Cluster Randomized Controlled Trial," *International Journal of Behavioral Nutrition and Physical Activity* 11 (2014): 10; U. Kinnunen, T. Feldt, J. de Bloom, and K. Korpela, "Patterns of Daily Energy Management at Work: Relations to Employee Well-Being and Job Characteristics," *International Archives of Occupational and Environmental Health* 88, no. 8 (2015): 1077–86; G. A. Nix, R. M. Ryan, J. B. Manly, and E. L. Deci, "Revitalization Through Self-Regulation: The Effects of Autonomous and Controlled Motivation on Happiness and Vitality," *Journal of Experimental Social Psychology* 35 (1999): 266–84.

8. Portions of this story are from Ms. Mullins's story told on *The Moth,* December 2, 2014, www.themoth.org.

9. J. Natour, L. A. Cazotti, L. H. Ribeiro, A. S. Baptista, and A. Jones, "Pilates Improves Pain, Function and Quality of Life in Patients with Chronic Low Back Pain: A Randomized Controlled Trail," *Clinical Rehabilitation* 29, no. 1 (2015): 59–68; B. S. Cheema, T. B. Davies, M. Stewart, S. Papalia, and E. Atlantis, "The Feasibility and Effectiveness of High-Intensity Boxing Training Versus Moderate-Intensity Brisk Walking in Adults with Abdominal Obesity: A Pilot Study," *BMC Sports Science, Medicine and Rehabilitation* 7, no. 3 (2015).

10. H. I. Catcher, H. R. Ferdowsian, V. J. Hoover, J. L. Cohen, and N. D. Barnard, "A Worksite Vegan Nutrition Program Is Well-Accepted and Improves Health-

Related Quality of Life and Work Productivity," *Annals of Nutrition Metabolism* 56 (2010): 245–52.

11. L. Landaeta-Diaz, J. M. Fernandez, M. Da Silva-Grigoletto, D. Rosado-Alvarez, A. Gomez-Garduno, et al., "Mediterranean Diet, Moderate-to-High Intensity Training, and Health-Related Quality of Life in Adults with Metabolic Syndrome," *European Journal of Preventive Cardiology* 20, no. 4 (2013): 555–64.

12. K. Nabe-Nielsen, A. H. Garde, K. Albertsen, and F. Diderichsen, "The Moderating Effect of Work-Time Influence on the Effect of Shift Work: A Prospective Cohort Study," *International Archive of Occupational and Environmental Health* 84 (2011): 551–59; L. Barber, M. J. Grawitch, and D. C. Munz, "Are Better Sleepers More Engaged Workers? A Self-Regulatory Approach to Sleep Hygiene and Work Engagement," *Stress and Health* 29, no. 4 (2012): 307–316.

13. T. Roth, T. Roehrs, and R. Pies, "Insomnia, Pathophysiology, and Implications for Treatment," *Sleep Medicine Reviews* 11, no. 1 (2007): 71–79.

14. P. La Cour and M. Petersen, "Effects of Mindfulness Meditation on Chronic Pain: A Randomized Controlled Trial," *Pain Medicine* 16, no. 4 (2015): 641–652; J. Halpern, M. Cohen, G. Kennedy, J. Reece, C. Cahan, and A. Baharav, "Yoga for Improving Sleep Quality and Quality of Life for Older Adults," *Alternative Therapies in Health and Medicine* 20, no. 3 (2014): 37–46.

15. L. O. Bygren, G. Weissglas, B. M. Wikström, B. B. Konlaan, A. Grjibovski, A. B. Karlsson, S. O. Andersson, and M. Sjöström, "Cultural Participation and Health: A Randomized Controlled Trial Among Medical Care Staff," *Psychosomatic Medicine* 71, no. 4 (2009): 469–73.

16. Direct analysis of MIDUS II (Midlife in the United States), a national sample of Americans aged twenty-five to seventy-four, from 2004 to 2006.

CHAPTER 7: WILLPOWER

1. W. C. Fields, quoted in F. R. Shapiro, *The Yale Book of Quotations,* section W. C. Fields (New Haven: Yale Univ. Press, 2006): 256.

2. T. R. Schlam, N. L. Wilson, Y. Shoda, W. Mischel, and O. Ayduk. "Preschoolers' Delay of Gratification Predicts Their Body Mass 30 Years Later," *The Journal of Pediatrics* 162, no. 1 (2012): 90–93; T. E. Moffitt, L. Arseneault, D. Belsky, et al., "A Gradient of Childhood Self-Control Predicts Health, Wealth, and Public Safety," *Proceedings of the National Academy of Science USA* 108, no. 7 (2011): 2693–98.

3. H. S. Decker, *Freud, Dora, and Vienna 1900* (New York: Free Press, 1991): 173.

4. F. Dostoevsky, *Winter Notes on Summer Impressions,* trans. David Patterson (Evanston, IL: Northwestern Univ. Press, 1997); 49.

5. D. J. Den Boer, G. Kok, H. J. Hospers, F. Gerards, and V. J. Strecher, "Health Education Strategies for Attributional Retraining and Self-Efficacy Improvement," *Health Education Research* 6, no. 2 (1991): 239–48.

6. R. F. Baumeister and J. Tierney, *Willpower: Rediscovering the Greatest Human Strength* (New York: Penguin Press, 2011): 7.

7. Y. Cornil and P. Chandon, "From Fan to Fat? Vicarious Losing Increases Unhealthy Eating, but Self-Affirmation Is an Effective Remedy," *Psychological Science* 24, no. 10 (2013): 1936–46.

8. B. Shiv and A. Fedorikhin, "Heart and Mind in Conflict: The Interplay of Affect and Cognition in Consumer Decision Making," *Journal of Consumer Research* 26, no. 3 (1999): 278.

9. O. Sacks, *The Man Who Mistook His Wife for a Hat and Other Clinical Tales* (New York: Touchstone, 1985): 97.

10. Cornil and Chandon, "From Fan to Fat?," 1936–46.

11. A. Burson, J. Crocker, and D. Mischkowski, "Two Types of Value-Affirmation: Implications for Self-Control Following Social Exclusion," *Social Psychological and Personality Science* 3, no. 4 (2012): 510–16.

12. X. Sun, X. Dai, T. Yang, H. Song, J. Yang, J. Bai, and L. Zhang "Effects of Mental Resilience on Neuroendocrine Hormones Level Changes Induced by Sleep Deprivation in Servicemen," *Endocrine* 47 (2014): 884–88.

13. R. C. Meldrum, J. C. Barnes, and C. Hay, "Sleep Deprivation, Low Self-Control, and Delinquency: A Test of the Strength Model of Self-Control," *Journal of Youth and Adolescence* 44, no. 2 (2015): 465–77.

14. D. J. Taylor, K. E. Vatthauer, A. D. Bramoweth, C. Ruggero, and B. Roane, "The Role of Sleep in Predicting College Academic Performance: Is It a Unique Predictor?" *Behavior Sleep Medicine* 11, no. 3 (2013): 159–72.

15. C. Yusainy and C. Lawrence, "Brief Mindfulness Induction Could Reduce Aggression After Depletion," *Consciousness and Cognition* 33 (2015): 125–34; D. Clark, Schumann, and Mostofsky, "Mindful Movement and Skilled Attention," *Frontiers in Human Neuroscience* 9 (2015): 297; S. M. Miller and R. E. Taylor-Piliae, "Effects of Tai Chi on Cognitive Function in Community-Dwelling Older Adults: A Review," *Geriatric Nursing* 35 (2014): 9–19.

16. P. La Cour and M. Petersen, "Effects of Mindfulness Meditation on Chronic Pain: A Randomized Controlled Trial. *Pain Medicine* 16, no. 4 (2014): 641–652.

17. B. K. Holzel, J. Carmody, M. Vangel, C. Congleton, S. M. Yerramsetti, T. Gard,

and S. W. Lazar, "Mindfulness Practice Leads to Increases in Regional Brain Gray Matter Density," *Psychiatry Research: Neuroimaging* 191 (2011): 36–43.

18. A. K. Converse, E. O. Ahlers, B. G. Travers, and R. J. Davidson, "Tai Chi Training Reduces Self-Report of Inattention in Healthy Young Adults," *Frontiers in Human Neuroscience* 8 (2014): 13.

19. C. C. Chang and Y. C. Lin, "Physical Activity and Food Consumption: The Moderating Role of Individual Dieting Tendency, *Journal of Health Psychology* 20, no. 5 (2015): 490–99.

20. K. McGonigal, "The Science of Willpower," *IDEA Fitness Journal,* June 2008, www.ideafit.com/fitness-library/science-willpower-0.

21. M. A. Runco, "Creativity," *Annual Review of Psychology* 55 (2004): 657–87.

22. D. Wei, J. Yang, W. Li, K. Wang, Q. Zhang, J. Quiz, "Increased Resting Functional Connectivity of the Medial Prefrontal Cortex in Creativity by Means of Cognitive Stimulation," *Cortex* 51 (2014): 92–102.

23. A. Fink, M. Benedek, et al., "Training of Verbal Creativity Modulates Brain Activity in Regions Associated with Language- and Memory-Related Demands," *Human Brain Mapping* 36, no. 10 (2015): 4104–15.

24. J. A. Arai and L. A. Feig, "Long-Lasting and Transgenerational Effects of an Environmental Enrichment on Memory Formation," *Brain Research Bulletin* 85, nos. 1–2 (2011): 30–35.

25. M. T. Gailliot and R. F. Baumeister, "The Physiology of Willpower: Linking Blood Glucose to Self-Control," *Personality and Social Psychology Review* 11, no. 4 (2007): 303–27.

CHAPTER 8: SLEEP

1. Jeff Warren, *The Head Trip: Adventures on the Wheel of Consciousness* (New York: Random House, 2007).

2. Warren, *The Head Trip*, 74.

3. S. S. Campbell and P. J. Murphy, "The Nature of Spontaneous Sleep Across Adulthood," *Journal of Sleep Research* 16, no. 1 (2007): 24–32.

4. S. Freud, *The Interpretation of Dreams* (New York: Basic Books, 1995).

5. Hans Eysenck, *Decline and Fall of the Freudian Empire* (New York: Viking Press, 1985): 208.

6. Warren, *The Head Trip*, 38.

CHAPTER 9: PRESENCE

1. Steve Jobs, quoted in W. Isaacson, *Steve Jobs* (New York: Simon & Schuster, 2011).

2. J. Kabat-Zinn, *Mindfulness for Beginners: Reclaiming the Present Moment—And Your Life* (Boulder, CO: Sounds True, 2012): 1.

3. M. Wittmann, S. Otten, E. Schotz, A. Sarikaya, et al., "Subjective Expansion of Extended Time-Spans in Experienced Meditators," *Frontiers in Psychology* 5 (2015): 1–9.

4. La Cour and Petersen, "Effects of Mindfulness Meditation on Chronic Pain," 641–52.

5. Y. Y. Tang, M. I. Posner, M. K. Rothbart, and N. D. Volkow, "Circuitry of Self-Control and Its Role in Reducing Addiction," *Trends in Cognitive Sciences,* July 13, 2015.

6. J. C. Ong, R. Manber, Z. Segal, Y. Zia, S. Shapiro, and J. K. Wyatt "A Randomized Controlled Trial of Mindfulness Meditation for Chronic Insomnia," *Sleep* 37, no. 9 (2014): 1553–63.

7. S. N. Katterman, B. M. Kleinman, M. M. Hood, L. M. Nackers, and J. A. Corsica. "Mindfulness Meditation as an Intervention for Binge Eating, Emotional Eating, and Weight Loss: A Systematic Review," *Eating Behaviors* 15, no. 2 (2014): 197–204.

8. M. Baas, B. Nevicka, and F. S. Ten Velden. "Specific Mindfulness Skills Differentially Predict Creative Performance," *Personality and Social Psychology Bulletin* 40 no. 9 (2014): 1092–1106.

9. E. M. Seppala, J. B. Nitschke, D. L. Tudorascu, A. Hayes, M. R. Goldstein, D. T. Nguyen, D. Perlman, and R. J. Davidson. "Breathing-Based Meditation Decreases Posttraumatic Stress Disorder Symptoms in U.S. Military Veterans: A Randomized Controlled Longitudinal Study," *Journal of Traumatic Stress* 27, no. 4 (2014): 397–405.

10. W. B. Britton, J. R. Lindahl, B. R. Cahn, J. H. Davis, and R. E. Goldman, "Awakening Is Not a Metaphor: The Effects of Buddhist Meditation Practices on Basic Wakefulness," *Annals of the New York Academy of Science* 1307 (2014): 64–81.

11. X. Liu, J. Clark, D. Siskind, G. M. Williams, et al., "A Systematic Review and Meta-analysis of the Effects of Qigong and Tai Chi for Depressive Symptoms," *Complementary Therapies in Medicine* 23 (2015): 516–34.

12. J. Halpern, M. Cohen, G. Kennedy, J. Reece, C. Cahan, and A. Baharav, "Yoga for Improvement of Sleep Quality and Quality of Life for Older Adults," *Alternative Therapies* 20 no. 3 (2014): 37–46.

13. J. K. Kiecolt-Glaser, J. M. Bennett, R. Andridge, J. Peng, et al., "Yoga's Impact on Inflammation, Mood, and Fatigue in Breast Cancer Survivors: A Randomized Controlled Trial," *Journal of Clinical Oncology* 32 (2014): 1040–49.

14. Inflammation was measured by the production of proinflammatory cytokines interleukin-6 (IL-6), tumor necrosis factor alpha (TNF-alpha), and interleukin-1beta (IL-1beta).

15. J. Haidt, J. P. Seder, and S. Kesebir, "Hive Psychology, Happiness, and Public Policy," *Journal of Legal Studies* 37 (2008): S133–S156.

CHAPTER 10: ACTIVITY

1. Aristotle, *Nicomachean Ethics*, trans. Terence Irwin, 2nd ed. (Cambridge: Hackett Publishing Company, 1999): 15.

2. K. Oskvig, "Harder, Faster, Stronger—Better: Aristotle's Ethics and Physical Human Enhancement," *Journal of Evolution & Technology* 23, no. 1 (2013): 19–30.

3. "Physical Activity," Centers for Disease Control and Prevention, 2015, www.cdc.gov/physicalactivity/.

4. Aristotle, *Rhetoric,* ed. W. D. Ross, trans. W. Rhys Roberts (New York: Cosimo Classics, 2010): 19.

5. G. Samitz, M. Egger, and M. Zwahlen, "Domains of Physical Activity and All-Cause Mortality: Systematic Review and Dose-Response Meta-analysis of Cohort Studies," *International Journal of Epidemiology* 40 (2011): 1382–1400.

6. C. Drenowatz, G. A. Hand, M. Sagner, R. P. Shook, S. Burgess, and S. N. Blair, "The Prospective Association Between Different Types of Exercise and Body Composition," *Medicine & Science in Sports & Exercise* 47, no. 12 (2015): 2535–41.

7. M. O'Dougherty, A. Arikawa, B. Kaufman, M. S. Kurzer, and K. H. Schmitz, "Purposeful Exercise and Lifestyle Physical Activity in the Lives of Young Adult Women: Findings from a Diary Study," *Women & Health* 49, no. 8 (2009): 642–61.

8. Department of Health and Human Services, *Be Active Your Way: A Guide for Adults,* October 2008, http://health.gov/paguidelines/pdf/adultguide.pdf.

9. A. Biswas, P. I. Oh, G. E. Faulkner, et al., "Sedentary Time and Its Association with Risk for Disease Incidence, Mortality, and Hospitalization in Adults," *Annals of Internal Medicine* 162 (2015): 123–32.

10. M. Segar, J. S. Eccles, and C. R. Richardson, "Type of Physical Activity Goal

Influences Participation in Healthy Midlife Women," *Women's Health Issues* 18 (2008): 281–91.

11.   M. Segar, D. Spruijt-etz, and S. Nolen-Hoeksema, "Body-Shape Motives Are Associated with Decreased Physical Activity Participation Among Midlife Women," *Sex Roles* 54, nos. 3/4 (2006): 175–87.

CHAPTER 11: CREATIVITY

1.   F. Nietzsche, *Philosophical Writings,* ed. R. Grimm and C. Molina y Vedia (New York: Continuum, 1997): 38.

2.   E. Hirsch, *How to Read a Poem* (Orlando, FL: Harcourt, 1999).

3.   E. Hirsch, www.artandhealing.org quoted in "Can Art Be Medicine?"

4.   K. J. Petrie, I. Fontanilla, M. G. Thomas, R. J. Booth, and J. W. Pennebaker, "Effect of Written Emotional Expression on Immune Function in Patients with Human Immunodeficiency Virus Infection: A Randomized Trial," *Psychosomatic Medicine* 66 (2004): 272–75; R. J. Davidson and B. S. McEwen. "Social Influences on Neuroplasticity: Stress and Interventions to Promote Well-Being," *Nature Neuroscience* 15, no. 5 (2013): 689–95.

5.   B. P. Chapman, K. Fiscella, I. Kawachi, P. Duberstein, and P. Muennig, "Emotion Suppression and Mortality Risk over a 12-Year Follow-Up," *Journal of Psychosomatic Research* 75, no. 4 (2013): 381–85.

6.   B. B. Konlaan, N. Bjorby, L. O. Bygren, G. Weissglas, L. G. Karlsson, and M. Widmark, "Attendance at Cultural Events and Physical Exercise and Health: A Randomized Controlled Study," *Public Health* 114 (2000): 316–19; T. W. Puetz, C. A. Morley, and M. P. Herring, "Effects of Creative Arts Therapies on Psychological Symptoms and Quality of Life in Patients with Cancer," *JAMA Internal Medicine* 173, no. 11 (2013): 960–69.

7.   R. May, *The Courage To Create* (New York: W. W. Norton, 1975): 15–16.

8.   Aristotle, *Politics,* VIII: 7; 1341b 35–1342a 8.

9.   L. Taruffi and S. Koelsch, "The Paradox of Music-Evoked Sadness: An Online Survey," *PLOS ONE* 9, no. 10 (2014): e110490.

10.   M. E. Sachs, A. Damasio, and A. Habibi, "The Pleasures of Sad Music: A Systematic Review," *Frontiers in Human Neuroscience* 9 (2015): 404.

11.   E. Brattico, V. Alluri, B. Bogert, T. Jacobsen, N. Vartiainen, S. Nieminen, et al., "A Functional MRI Study of Happy and Sad Emotions in Music with and Without Lyrics," *Frontiers in Psychology* 2 (2011): 1–16, 308.

12. B. Sharkey, "Lars von Trier's 'Melancholia' Is—Gasp—Hopeful," *Los Angeles Times,* November 11, 2011.

13. M. Montgomery and C. Montgomery, *Hubert Invents the Wheel* (New York: Walker & Company, 2005).

14. D. Adams, *The Hitchhiker's Guide to the Galaxy* (New York: Harmony Books, 1979).

15. Found at Famous Last Words, http://web.mit.edu/randy/www/words.html.

16. M. Bellomo, *Toys & Prices: The World's Best Toys Price Guide,* 19th ed. (Iola, WI: Krause Publications): 167.

17. M. Zager, *Music Production: For Producers, Composers, Arrangers, and Students,* 2nd ed. (Toronto: The Scarecrow Press, 2012): 222.

18. "Best-Sellers Initially Rejected," *LitRejections,* www.litrejections.com/best-sellers-initially-rejected/.

19. D. Oshinsky, "No Thanks, Mr. Nabokov," Sunday Book Review, *New York Times,* September 9, 2007.

20. R. Asri, "7 Famous Books That Were Passed Over by Publishers," *Arts.Mic,* August 3, 2013, http://mic.com/articles/57389/7-famous-books-that-were-passed-over-by-publishers#.gvCcsJhv0.

21. E. Degas, *The Notebooks of Edgar Degas,* trans. T. Reff (Oxford: Oxford Univ. Press, 1976).

22. C. G. Jung, *Memories, Dreams, Reflections* (New York: Vintage Books, 1961).

23. C. G. Jung, *Psychological Types,* trans. H. Read, M. Fordham, and G. Adler, *The Collected Works of C. G. Jung,* vol. 6 (New York: Routledge, 1991): para. 757, 448.

24. Nietzsche, *The Gay Science,* 232–33.

25. J. Marsden, D. Budden, H. Craig, and P. Moscato, "Language Individuation and Marker Words: Shakespeare and His Maxwell's Demon," *PLOS ONE* 8, no. 6 (2013): e66813.

26. Nietzsche, *The Gay Science,* 232–33.

27. S. Liu, et al. "Brain Activity and Connectivity During Poetry Composition: Toward a Multidimensional Model of the Creative Process," *Human Brain Mapping* 36 (2015): 3351–72.

28. M. Baas, B. Nevicka, and F. S. Ten Velden, "Specific Mindfulness Skills Differentially Predict Creative Performance," *Personality and Social Psychology Bulletin* 40, no. 9 (2014): 1092–1106.

29. C. Hawthorne, "Michael Graves Dies at 80; Pioneering Figure in Postmodern Architecture," *Los Angeles Times,* March 12, 2015, www.latimes.com/local/obituaries/la-me-michael-graves-20150313-story.html.

CHAPTER 12: EATING

1. J. Confino, "Zen Master Thich Nhat Hanh: Only Love Can Save Us from Climate Change," *The Guardian,* January 21, 2013.

2. S. Danzinger, J. Levav, and L. Avnaim-Pesso, "Extraneous Factors in Judicial Decisions," *Proceedings of the National Academy of Science* 108, no. 17 (2011): 6889–92.

3. National Public Radio, "'Fast And Slow': Pondering the Speed of Thought," an interview with Daniel Kahneman, October 19, 2011.

4. D. D. Clark and L. Sokoloff, "Circulation and Energy Metabolism of the Brain," in *Basic Neurochemistry: Molecular, Cellular and Medical Aspects,* ed. G. J. Siegel, B. W. Agranoff, R. W. Albers, S. K. Fisher, and M. D. Uhler (Philadelphia: Lippincott, 1999): 637–70.

5. M. E. Raichle and D. A. Gusnard, "Appraising the Brain's Energy Budget," *PNAS* 99, no. 16 (2002): 10237–39.

6. Baumeister and Tierney, *Willpower.*

7. M. T. Gailliot and R. F. Baumeister, "The Physiology of Willpower: Linking Blood Glucose to Self-Control," *Personality and Social Psychology Review* 11, no. 4 (2007): 303–27.

8. S. N. Bleich, J. A. Wolfson, S. Vine, and Y. C. Wang, "Diet-Beverage Consumption and Caloric Intake Among U.S. Adults, Overall and by Body Weight," *American Journal of Public Health* 104, no. 3 (2014): e72–e78.

9. D. Lieberman, *The Story of the Human Body* (New York: Pantheon, 2013).

10. I. Shai, D. Schwarzfuchs, Y. Henkin, et al., "Weight Loss with a Low-Carbohydrate, Mediterranean or Low-Fat Diet. *The New England Journal of Medicine* 359, no. 3 (2008), 229–41.

11. H. I. Catcher, H. R. Ferdowsian, V. J. Hoover, J. L. Cohen, and N. D. Barnard, "A Worksite Vegan Nutrition Program Is Well-Accepted and Improves Health-Related Quality of Life and Work Productivity," *Annals of Nutrition Metabolism* 56 (2010): 245–52.

12. B. Wansink, J. E. Painter, and K. van Ittersum, "Descriptive Menu Labels' Effect on Sales," *Cornell Hotel and Restaurant Administration Quarterly* 42 (2001): 68–72.

13. B. Wansink, K. van Ittersum, and J. E. Painter, "Ice Cream Illusions: Bowls, Spoons, and Self-Served Portion Sizes," *American Journal of Preventive Medicine* 31, no. 3 (2006): 240–43.

14. B. Wansink, *Mindless Eating: Why We Eat More than We Think* (New York: Bantam, 2006).

15. T. S. Conner, K. L. Brookie, A. C. Richardson, and M. A. Polak, "On Carrots and Curiosity: Eating Fruit and Vegetables Is Associated with Greater Flourishing in Daily Life," *British Journal of Health Psychology* 20, no. 4 (2015): 413–27.

16. F. Depeint, W. R. Bruce, N. Shangari, R. Mehta, and P. J. O'Brien, "Mitochondrial Function and Toxicity: Role of the B Vitamin Family on Mitochondrial Energy Metabolism," *Chemico-Biological Interactions* 163, no. 1 (2006): 94–112.

17. Aristotle, *Nicomachean Ethics,* ed. S. Broadie and C. Rowe (Oxford: Oxford Univ. Press, 2002), 112.

18. Edgar Saltus, *Oscar Wilde: An Idler's Impression* (Chicago: Brothers of the Book, 1917): 19.

CHAPTER 13: SAILING THROUGH STORMS

1. David Foster Wallace, *This Is Water: Some Thoughts, Delivered on a Significant Occasion, about Living a Compassionate Life* (New York: Little, Brown, and Company, 2009): 53–55.

2. From her story told at the Aspen Ideas Festival, 2015.

3. A. Feder, A. Ahmad, E. J. Lee, J. E. Morgan, R. Singh, B. W. Smith, S. M. Southwick, and D. S. Charney, "Coping and PTSD Symptoms in Pakistani Earthquake Survivors: Purpose in Life, Religious Coping and Social Support," *Journal of Affective Disorders* 147 (2013): 156–63.

4. Y. Jin, J. Xu, H. Liu, and D. Liu, "Posttraumatic Stress Disorder and Posttraumatic Growth Among Adult Survivors of Wenchuan Earthquake after 1 Year: Prevalence and Correlates," *Archives of Psychiatric Nursing* 28 (2014): 67–73.

5. J. Chen, X. Zhou, M. Zeng, and X. Wu, "Post-traumatic Stress Symptoms and Post-traumatic Growth: Evidence from a Longitudinal Study Following an Earthquake Disaster," *PLOS ONE* 10, no. 6 (2015): e0127241.

6. W. Duan and G. Penfei, "Association Between Virtues and Posttraumatic Growth: Preliminary Evidence from a Chinese Community Sample after Earthquakes," *PeerJ* 3 (2015): e883. Note: The authors use different terms for energy and willpower. Energy is called "vitality," and willpower is called "cautiousness" (which includes concepts such as self-regulation, perseverance, judgment, and prudence).

7. Y. Kyutoku, et al., "Cognitive and Psychological Reactions of the General Population Three Months after the 2011 Tohoku Earthquake and Tsunami," *PLOS ONE* 7, no. 2 (2012): e31014.

8. K. Taku, A. Can, R. G. Tedeschi, and L. G. Calhoun, "Core Beliefs Shaken by an Earthquake Correlate with Posttraumatic Growth," *Psychological Trauma: Theory, Research, Practice, and Policy* 7, no. 6 (May 25, 2015): 563–69.

9. A. Crowell, E. Page-Gould, and B. J. Schmeichel, "Self-Affirmation Breaks the Link Between the Behavioral Inhibition System and the Threat-Potentiated Startle Response," *Emotion* 15, no. 2 (2015): 146–50.

10. C. M. van Reekum, et al., "Individual Differences in Amygdala and Ventromedial Prefrontal Cortex Activity Are Associated with Evaluation Speed and Psychological Well-Being," *Journal of Cognitive Neuroscience* 19 (2007): 237–48.

11. S. M. Schaefer, J. Morozink-Boyland, C. M. van Reekum, R. C. Lapate, C. J. Norris, C. D. Ryff, and R. J. Davidson, "Purpose in Life Predicts Better Emotional Recovery from Negative Stimuli," *PLOS ONE* 8, no. 11 (2013): e80329.

12. B. W. Smith, et al., "The Role of Resilience and Purpose in Life in Habituation to Heat and Cold Pain," *The Journal of Pain* 10, no. 5 (2009): 493–500.

13. E. Puterman and E. Epel, "An Intricate Dance: Life Experience, Multisystem Resiliency, and Rate of Telomere Decline Throughout the Lifespan," *Social and Personality Psychology Compass* 6, no. 11 (2012): 807–25.

14. S. Kallem, et al., "Shift-and-Persist: A Protective Factor for Elevated BMI Among Low Socioeconomic Status Children," *Obesity* 21 (2013): 1759–63.

15. E. Chen E, et al., "Resilience in Low-Socioeconomic-Status Children with Asthma: Adaptations to Stress," *Journal of Allergy and Clinical Immunology* 128 (2011): 970–76.

16. E. Chen, K. C. McLean, and G. E. Miller, "Shift-and-Persist Strategies: Associations with Socioeconomic Status and the Regulation of Inflammation Among Adolescents and Their Parents," *Psychosomatic Medicine* 77 (2015): 371–82. Remember from chapter 2 that inflammation is associated with a wide range of diseases.

17. Countries with far lower averages include Germany, the Netherlands, China, and Russia. The United States falls slightly lower than average.

18. M. A. Ali, "Somalian Solution to the Perilous Exodus," Op-Ed, *New York Times,* May 11, 2015.

19. A. P. Teques, G. B. Carrera, J. P. Ribeiro, P. Teques, and G. L. Ramon, "The Importance of Emotional Intelligence and Meaning in Life in Psycho-Oncology," *Psycho-Oncology,* August 10, 2015.

20. M. O. Owolabi, "Consistent Determinants of Post-stroke Health-Related Quality of Life Across Diverse Cultures: Berlin-Ibadan Study," *Acta Neurologica Scandinavica* 128, no. 5 (2013): 311–20.

21. C. M. van Leeuwen, Y. Edelaar-Peeters, C. Peter, A. M. Stiggelbout, and M. W.

Post, "Psychological Factors and Mental Health in Persons with Spinal Cord Injury: An Exploration of Change or Stability," *Journal of Rehabilitation Medicine*
47, no. 6 (2015): 531–31.

22. M. Senthilingam, E. Pietersen, R. McNerney, J. Te Riele, P. Sedres, R. Wilson,
and K. Dheda, "Lifestyle, Attitudes and Needs of Uncured XDR-TB Patients
Living in the Communities of South Africa: A Qualitative Study," *Tropical
Medicine & International Health* 20, no. 9 (2015): 1155–61.

23. R. S. Farber, M. L. Kern, and E. Brusilovsky, "Integrating the ICF with Positive
Psychology: Factors Predicting Role Participation for Mothers with Multiple
Sclerosis," *Rehabilitation Psychology* 60, no. 2 (2015): 169–78.

24. S. C. Danhauer, et al., "A Longitudinal Investigation of Posttraumatic Growth
in Adult Patients Undergoing Treatment for Leukemia," *Journal of Clinical Psychology in Medical Settings* 20, no. 1 (2013): 13–24.

25. Ram Dass, quoted in E. Lesser, *Broken Open: How Difficult Times Can Help Us
Grow* (New York: Random House, 2004).

CHAPTER 14: AN EXCELLENT SAILOR

1. L. Annaeus Seneca, *On the Shortness of Life,* trans. J. W. Basore, Loeb Classical Library (London: William Heinemann, 1932), found at Corpus Scriptorum
Latinorum, a Digital Library of Latin Literature, www.forumromanum.org/
literature/seneca_younger/brev_e.html.

2. S. Hawking and L. Mlodinow, *The Grand Design* (New York: Random House,
2010): 5.

3. Nietzsche, *The Gay Science,* 335.

4. K. Eagan, E. B. Stolzenberg, J. J. Ramirez, M. C. Aragon, M. R. Suchard, and
S. Hurtado, *The American Freshman: National Norms Fall 2014* (Los Angeles:
Higher Education Research Institute, UCLA, 2014).

5. J. Helliwell, R. Layard, and J. Sachs, eds., *World Happiness Report* (New York:
Sustainable Development Solutions Network, 2012).

6. B. Russell, *On Education: Especially in Early Childhood* (New York: Routledge,
2003): 22.

7. L. Annaeus Seneca, *L. Annaeus Seneca, Minor Dialogs Together with the Dialog
on Clemency,* trans. A. Stewart (London: George Bell and Sons, 1900), 162–203.

8. Lesser, *Broken Open.*

9. Shaw, *Man and Superman,* 7.

Index

Abdul-Jabbar, Kareem, 64
Abraham and Isaac story, 89
activity: Aristotle on benefits of, 163, 165; description and types of, 167–71; getting started, 169–71; as good for sleep, 140; how physical environments can shape your, 172–73; Mike Mosallam's story on benefits of, 165–67, 169, 170, 172, 173–74; simple tips to increase your, 173–77; as source of energy, 110, 126, 239; as source of willpower, 124–25, 239; studies on health benefits of, 110, 169, 170–71
activity exercises: aerobic, 168, 169; balance, 168; flexibility, 168; resistance, 168, 169
Adams, Douglas, 187–88
ADHD (attention-deficit/hyperactivity disorder), 120, 121, 124
adolescents: brain research on eudaimonic versus hedonic decision making by, 31–32; research findings on depressive symptoms and eudaimonic vs. hedonic reward systems of, 32. *See also* children
aerobic exercise, 168, 169
afterlife beliefs, 92–94
age differences in values, 49
agency. *See* human agency
AIDS epidemic, 51, 221
AIDS orphan, 224
Ailey, Alvin, 184
Alchemist, The (Coelho), 96–97
alcohol consumption: affirming values to reduce, 53; blood glucose decreased by, 206; improving sleep by less, 138, 139; special secret monkish tip on meditating before allowing a drink, 162

alcohol rehab, 15, 16
Alexander the Great, 23, 47, 165
Ali, Mohamed Abdulkadir, 232–33
All-American Muslim (TLC series), 166
Allen, Woody, 50
Also sprach Zarathustra (Strauss), 45
altruistic behaviors: "otherish," 69; studies of animal, 67–68; study findings on adult reward systems undermined children's, 68
Alzheimer's Disease, 14, 16
ambition virtue, 47
American College of Sports Medicine, 167, 169
amygdala, 231
anarchy, 71
Andrews, Julie, 17
animals: sleep patterns of, 132; studies on altruistic behavior by, 67–68
Apollo (Greek god), 24
Appalachian Trail speed record, 61–62
appreciation expression, 183–85
Arinaitwe, James, 224–25, 232
Aristotle: on benefits of activity, 163, 165, 168; "best purpose" meaning of his name, 33; on eudaimonia happiness versus "hedonia" happiness, 26–27, 172; examination and reason focus of, 77; on getting "innocent joy" from said music, 184; Hawking's dismissal of, 21; his observations on individuals with eudaimonia, 30; on nature of being happy, 101; on obtaining the virtues of eudaimonic life from emulation of worthy people, 50; as student of Plato and teacher to Alexander the Great, 23, 47;

personal legend: comprehending our, 94–97;
Julia's continued, 97

Pharr Davis, Jennifer: attempting to break
the Appalachian Trail speed record,
61–62; inspired by her husband Brew,
62; reaching success by transcending
her purpose for hiking, 63–64

Philip Morris, 73

philosophy: Hawking's on the death of,
21–22, 288; Hindu, 69, 93, 147–48;
Krauss on superiority of science over,
22–23, 28; remember to HANDLE
WITH CARE, 46–47

photovoice project (South Africa), 51–52

physical activity. *See* activity

Picasso, Pablo, 88, 90

Plato, 23, 165

Play It Again, Sam (film), 50

political leaning values, 49

"polyphasic" sleep patterns, 134

Potting Shed, The (Greene), 85

presence: description and examples of,
148–50; movement practices to
achieve, 154–55; movement practices to
increase, 154–55; power of the hive on,
156–57; as source of energy, 111, 126,
239; as source of willpower, 124, 126,
239; Steve Jobs on, 143; tips for increasing your, 159–62. *See also* meditation;
mindfulness

Priyadarshi, Tenzin, 145–47, 148

prostate-specific antigen (PSA) level, 76

"protestant ethic" values, 47

psychology: Jung's individuation, 190;
Maslow's humanistic, 63; on the "white
bear" effect, 116

PTSD (post-traumatic stress disorder):
earthquake studies on survivor, 228;
studies on healing power of art expression on, 182; study on "breathing meditation" to decrease, 150. *See also* stress

public health studies: cohorts used in, 13;
efforts to avoid mistaking correlation
for causation in, 13–14; on the power
of values to affirm positive health
behaviors, 52–53

Pulp Fiction (film), 86–87

purpose as a goal: creativity generated

through, 186–87; the headstone test to
assess your goals and, 43–44, 57, 93–94;
Jerry Hirsch's embrace of, 43–44;
overview of the, 40–43; setting big and
lofty goals for your, 41; taking different
roles for achieving different goals and,
41–43

purpose as a value: affirmation through,
52–53; age differences in, 49; Aristotle
on the most valuable of virtues, 47;
Benjamin Franklin's list of desired
values, 47; cultural norms limiting our
agency to create our, 44–45; emulating
worthy people to obtain worthy, 50–52;
Falk's study of value affirmation in
the vmPFC, 54–55; gender differences
in, 48–49; human agency giving us
the ability to choose what we value,
44; Nietzsche's camel into lion allegory on creating our own, 45, 47, 109;
political leanings and associated, 49;
"protestant ethic" and capitalism, 47;
self-determination to make decisions
based on one's, 107–9; social and personal factors that impact our, 49; "Why
Does Writing about Important Values
Reduce Defensiveness?" study on, 55;
World Values Survey on cultural differences in, 48, 232

Purpose Driven Life, The (Warren), 87

purposeful people: Aimee Mullins, 108–9,
165, 243; Esther Ngumbi, 222–24,
230; Henry Nyombi, 225–27, 230, 243;
how their resilience is reinforced by
purpose, 227–33; James Arinaitwe,
224–25, 232; Mike Mosallam, 165–67,
169, 170, 172, 173–74; positive "breaking open" effect shared by, 233

purpose in life: creativity generated through,
186–87; don't confuse meaning in life
with, 56; giving life Technicolor, 7, 9;
Google searches on, 242; having hope
as part of, 232; as a higher-order goal,
40–44; imagining it as a medication with
similar health benefits, 16–17; Jim Loehr
on the dynamic activity of being aligned
with your, 103–4; Julia's postmortem
message on having a, 5–6, 9;